MAN IN HIS RELATIONSHIPS

Founded by C. K. Ogden

The International Library of Psychology

PSYCHOLOGY AND RELIGION
In 6 Volumes

MAN IN HIS RELATIONSHIPS

Edited by H WESTMANN

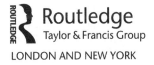

LONDON AND NEW YORK

First published in 1955
by Routledge
2 Park Square, Milton Park, Abingdon, Oxfordshire OX14 4RN
711 Third Avenue, New York, NY 10017

First issued in paperback 2014

Routledge is an imprint of the Taylor and Francis Group, an informa business

British Library Cataloguing in Publication Data
A CIP catalogue record for this book
is available from the British Library

Man in His Relationships
ISBN 0415-21115-8
Psychology and Religion: 6 Volumes
ISBN 0415-21133-6
The International Library of Psychology: 204 Volumes
ISBN 0415-19132-7

ISBN 13: 978-1-138-87573-9 (pbk)
ISBN 13: 978-0-415-21115-4 (hbk)

Contents

Editor's Note

MAN IN HIS RELATIONSHIPS was the theme of the tenth Present Question Conference which was held at Lady Margaret Hall, Oxford in July 1954.

The initial idea of Present Question was formulated in 1945 in the following terms:—

'The atomic bomb had not yet fallen on Hiroshima; the war was not yet over. There was the uneasy feeling that the agony of the past years did not produce a solution to our problem. What problem? Do we know it? Has our specialized approach to Life made us forget how to ask the right question? Can we expect to find a valid answer without having first asked the right question?

Can both Answer and Question be found by putting one fundamental problem in the centre, towards which, like the petals of a flower, each specialized field of human knowledge gives its contribution?'

Today, after ten years, we believe that we see more clearly that the fundamental human problem of modern society is in fact the integration of diversity of experience—the bridging of the gap between specialisms. Whether this problem shows itself in the difficulties of international co-operation, in labour management relations, in problems of local community life or in any of the varied fields exemplified in the different approaches to the theme of this book or to the subjects of former Conferences—fundamentally the problem for modern society seems to lie in *the need for communication between the varying specialized fields*. The satisfaction of this need is imperative if the society of the West is to remain responsible and free.

Editor's Note

While in most conferences dealing with the problems of modern society interest is concentrated on the subject-matter, the distinctive feature of Present Question is that it is concerned not so much with subject-matter—though subject-matter is dealt with at the highest level—as with the attempt, through the discussion of subject-matter, to *bring about communication*. Its whole emphasis is on fostering and deepening face-to-face discussion between those who represent diverse experience, as the most fruitful method of advancing the integration which is so essential to the whole future of modern society.

Secretariat,   H.W.
38-40 Beaumont Street,
London, W.1.

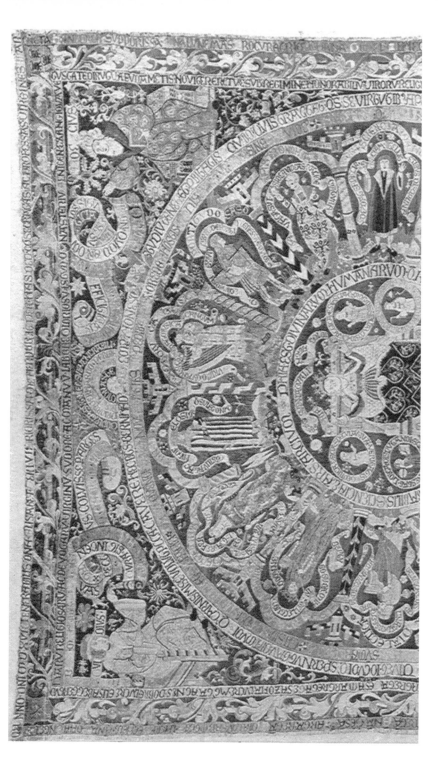

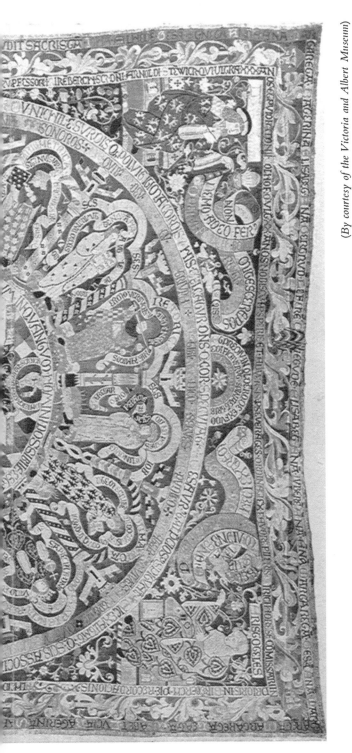

(By courtesy of the Victoria and Albert Museum)

The Heiningen Carpet (A.D. 1516) is a pictorial representation of the Present Question Idea. The carpet shows *Philosophia* surrounded by *Teorica, Practica, Loica, Mechanica,* and *Phisica,* forming the inner circle. The outer circle depicts various sciences and mental and moral qualities of man. In the four corners are seated four ancient philosophers: *Ovid, Boethius, Horace* and *Aristotle.* The carpet as a whole depicts the idea of the Anthropos; in whom "are gathered together one in all things", the primordial image of the potentially rounded completeness of personality.

Man in Relation to Himself

H. WESTMANN

Psychotherapist; Founder of the Present Question Conference

THE SOCIAL and cultural advance of man is directly related to the development of personality. This has been, and still is, a very slow and gradual affair. Even now, man has achieved only a limited awareness of himself as personality. At the very threshold of history our primitive ancestors lived in what Lévy-Bruhl has well described as a *participation mystique*, a mystical sharing, with Nature. At this stage there was still no clear differentiation in man's mind between himself and his environment. Only later, as man grew slowly towards an awareness of himself as personality, did it become possible for him to see both himself and the external world in relation to one another, and so to transcend his earlier containment within the dark forces of nature.

This growth of a sense of relatedness brought with it something else, the first stirrings of the scientific consciousness. For man, now beginning to be aware of himself, could begin to see nature as something 'other', as phenomena standing apart, which could be observed and investigated. But the differentiation of Man from Nature was, if I may so express it, only the permissive condition for the growth of true science. Something else was needed.

'It is quite clear to me', writes Professor John Baillie, 'that modern science could not have come into being until the ancient pagan conception of the natural world had given place to the Christian.'[1] The pagan world-view was largely atomistic. Each separate event was ruled by its own constellation of conditioning impulses. With the monotheism of the Old Testament came something new: the assertion of a creation by a God who was not only Creator but also Lawgiver to his creation. This belief predisposed man's mind to an enhanced empathy with the unitary character of the Universe, grounded in the faith that man is made in the image of the One God. The next step was taken with the Christianity of the New Testament—the mystery of God becoming man, and St. Paul's confident hope that 'in the dispensation of the fullness of times he might gather together in one all things'.

As time went on, however, the phenomenal achievements of science fostered a sense of human power and self-sufficiency that was the antithesis of Christian humility. Practical success was a heady and intoxicating draught. For Laplace in the eighteenth century, God had become an hypothesis which science no longer needed. Why indeed could not man himself become as God? Was he not the master in a mechanistic universe that human science could both explain and control?

The further development of science has itself exposed the hollowness of these pretensions. In the new climate of scientific thought, old certainties have become uncertain, and eternal truths have lost their timelessness. Perhaps the most important factor responsible for this change has been the virtual replacement of the observer-predictor attitude by the activity of the observer-participant. The ideal of the elimination of the person of the scientist from the process of experiment, so as to achieve the highest degree of objectivity, has had to be abandoned in one field after another. The gap between the observer and the observed system cannot any longer be kept open. Man himself is involved.

As long as he could persuade himself that he was looking at facts 'objectively', man felt secure. Now the indubitable 'fact' has again become a mystery. Pure objectivity is now seen to be pure illusion. The recognition of the observer's own involvement in what he is observing has again restored man's psyche to its central position in the scheme of things—to a

[1]*Natural Science and the Spiritual Life* (Oxford University Press).

position from which the scientists of earlier centuries hoped they had removed it forever.

Since man is potentially a unity and totality in himself, he is inescapably committed to the search for unity in the world of experience. This inner potentiality in man, that ever seeks to realize itself as a unity, is what I propose to call personality. The word personality is so important that I must try to define it as precisely as possible. But it is very difficult to circumscribe it by a definition, for personality is not a 'thing' but a living and developing system. We may describe it as an organic unity, an intimate fusion of what man is with everything he does. But man's actions depend not only on the conscious mind; they are conditioned in a high degree by the unconscious. His personality—the organic complex of thoughts, desires, impulses, actions and memories which make him what he is—embraces both conscious and unconscious elements, in perpetually changing interplay. As long as man is unaware of this close interrelation, he is only partially aware of himself as a personality. I believe, therefore, that the ground and aim of our human existence can be summed up as the achievement of a relationship of awareness to personality.

Such awareness is the precondition of our being able to function, either as a contributing and responding part of a greater whole, or as a personality in our own right. It is the integration of the unconscious with the conscious which in the end leads to awareness of true personality, awareness of the Self.

This Self cannot exist in isolation. It is only 'there', as it were, as the nodal point of a system of inter-relations to which every aspect of life's many-sided richness makes its contribution. The difficulty of conveying the true sense of this concept is obvious. The centre of personality is not something that can be observed and measured in the way that we observe and measure the behaviour of matter. And yet we are all to some degree aware of its meaning. Today people are beginning slowly to realize that there has been a shift from the centre, that modern man has become 'off centre'. Through identification with particular aspects of life at the expense of others, we have produced abstracts of man in many varieties. These go by such names as 'scientific man', 'economic man', 'political man' and the like.

3

In all this, there is a great danger, because a shifting away from the centre makes man less than himself; the false selves he creates cannot satisfy him. This is why in our present society there is so widespread a sense of meaninglessness about our existence. We have forgotten that our grandest challenge lies in the development of ourselves as full personalities. Instead we degrade personality to a means serving an end, and forget that personality is, as Professor Tillich has said[1], an end and purpose in itself. Man today suffers within his own soul the tyrannical rule of the part over the whole. The shifting of the Self, as the vital centre of personality, out to the periphery, and its identification with narrow specialisms, has led directly to the impersonality of modern life, has distorted personal relationships, and falsified our recognition of personal and collective responsibility.

But how can man be helped to achieve a sound relationship to himself and fulfil his eternal task of growth from potential to actual personality? In ancient times over the porch of the Delphic oracle were written the words 'Know Thyself'. Present-day psychology also attempts to approach the uncertainties of human existence through self-knowledge. Freud revived this ancient wisdom by looking at man mainly in his family relationships. For him, the whole process of the development of the psyche depended ultimately upon the integration of the child-parent relation. In Freud's view all cultural progress as well as the achievement of moral order, rested on this integration. Jung widened the psychological horizon to take in the whole inter-related range of human experience. Nevertheless, at the centre of both the Freudian and Jungian approaches to the psyche lies the notion of the growth and development of consciousness. The necessary condition of such growth is the development of personal awareness of two primary modes of human reaction: firstly, of the rôle of the instincts, and secondly of that of the archetypes. I propose to confine myself to the archetypes.

The word 'archetype' may sound strange to many ears, but it has an honourable history. Long before it became a fundamental concept in Analytical Psychology it was used by Ambrose and Tertullian. St. Augustine's 'principales formae'

[1] *The Protestant Era*, p. 129 ff.

4

is a rendering of the Greek 'archetypoi'. He writes: 'They themselves do not come into being or perish, but everything which does come into being and perishes is said to be formed according to them . . . These primary things are not only ideas, but are true, because they are eternal and because they remain the same and unchangeable. Through participation in them it happens that everything is what it is and how it is.' (*De Quaestionibus Octaginta Tribus. Q.46. De Ideas (Migne P.L.XL.)*)

Etymologically, the word 'archetype' is derived from the Greek words *arche*, first, foremost or chief; and *tupos*, a blow or the mark left by a blow, an impress or a mould. We are familiar with the first element in such words as archipelago, architect, archbishop; and with the second in type, typical and so on. The word 'Archetype', as used in Analytical Psychology, is perhaps best rendered as 'master pattern'. The archetypes are held to belong to man's remotest inheritance. They are patterns of behaviour through which his actions are unconsciously conditioned, and may therefore be regarded as *a priori* categories reaching back into levels of experience where man neither knows nor remembers.

It is difficult to explain the idea of the archetype in logical propositions, for its meaning can be fully grasped only through personal experience. I will, however, try to bring as much illumination to the question as I can by considering how the archetypes actually operate, first in imaginative artistic creation, and second in the activity of communication.

Let us then look first at the archetypes as *a priori* categories of the imagination. May I elucidate the meaning of this somewhat enigmatic formulation with a few quotations. In a recent lecture, Sir Kenneth Clark spoke of 'moments of vision', which alike in painting and poetry emerge with unpredictable vividness to dominate a whole work of art. He goes on to suggest that the clue to the compulsive, all-embracing character of these experiences may well be the feeling of self-discovery or self-identification that often accompanies them. The 'moment of vision' is related 'to something within us that already and forever exists'. This last phrase is from Coleridge. Here is the whole passage from which it is taken: 'In looking at objects . . . as at yonder moon dim glimmering through the dewy

5

pane, I seem rather to be seeking, as it were asking a symbolical language for something within me that forever and already exists, than observing anything new. Even when that latter is the case yet still I have always an obscure feeling, as if that new phenomenon were a dim awakening of a forgotten or hidden truth of my inner nature.'[1]

Let me add to this three more quotations. The first is from the English poet John Heath-Stubbs. He writes: 'The artist starts from an intuition of the underlying unity of the phenomena of the Universe which it is the goal of the scientist to establish. The artist unlooses archetypal and unconscious symbols the moral effect of which he cannot himself estimate . . . and it is in the imagination generally that we find the growing points of the human race and of society'[2]. And next a very important quotation from Sir Herbert Read: 'A sense of reality is a conquest, an advance from the chaos and confusion of an unintelligible world: a construction. The first order introduced into man's conception of the world was an aesthetic order— the order of ritual and myth. Later the intellect gradually made a selection of the totality—the part it can describe and measure —and gave it a more or less coherent unity, and called it science. The map is constantly enlarged: new details are filled in; but vast territories of space and time must still be marked "terra incognita". The sensibility plays like lightning over these dark abysses, and in the flashes gets a brief glimpse of the lineaments of this Unknown: the brief glimpse that is the artist's intuition, and which he then strives to communicate to us by the symbols he invents. That is the moment of originality—the moment in which we are made to realize the ethereal shimmering texture of music, the "shapes that haunt thought's wilderness", in poetry, the "beauty wrought out from within upon the flesh" of a painting. Poetry, painting, music—all these are arts or skills for raising the senses to that condition of insight, in which the world is not transfigured but in which for the first time some aspect of it is revealed, or made real, and thereby, for human eyes newly created, newly communicated'.[3]

[1]*Anima Poetae*, p. 136.
[2]*Question*, vol. 5, p. 123.
[3]*Sewanee Review*, October 1953.

And finally, as an illustration of archetypal expression in poetry, here are a few lines from 'Villanelle', by John Wain.[1]

> True oracles say more than they suppose.
> Your very dumbness makes your message clear.
> The clown may speak what silent Hamlet knows.
>
> A harmless droll is what the camera shows,
> The children's friend whom parents need not fear.
> True oracles say more than they suppose.
>
> In your fake world of frantic gag and pose
> We see our real despair come striding near.
> The clown may speak what silent Hamlet knows.

Henry Moore, Picasso, Chagall, among many others, picture in their work what are clearly archetypal experiences. Here too, we cannot help realizing that we are in the presence of 'dim awakenings of a forgotten or hidden truth of our inner nature'.

And now a few words on the Archetypes as modes of communication. Both art and science are essentially concerned with the communication of experience through symbols. Professor Ritchie goes so far as to say that 'the essential act of thought is symbolization'. After all, it is the same with thought as it is with spoken or written language, where every combination of sounds or letters stands for (or symbolizes) the experience that lies behind its meaning. Man, or more precisely the human psyche, is the channel through which deepest experience finds expression and communicates its essential quality. In other words, we may say that man is the medium through which life becomes conscious of itself.

Artistic creation is one of the highest expressions of communication. But in the creative work of the great artist, whether conveyed in words, music, colour or form, we recognize, no matter how infinitely varied the specific imagery may be, a universal character. The explanation lies in the universality of the archetypal content which infuses and gives form to the experience which the artist re-creates and communicates. Although the particular symbolism employed will vary from one culture to another, and from one artist to another, the

[1]*Images of To-morrow*, S.C.M. Press.

symbols necessarily illustrate a theme. The fact that they constitute 'variations on a theme' does not justify us in refusing to recognize that the theme itself is in the highest degree meaningful. We may sum this up by quoting C. G. Jung's unambiguous statement that 'the archetype is not the consequence of physical facts, but rather shows how physical facts are experienced by the soul'.

What holds true for art holds true also for communication between persons. We can experience in a relation with another person a kind of communication, almost of communion, which goes far beyond what is mediated by the physical senses alone. In such a relation we in fact comprehend the 'thou' in symbols. The validation of these symbols must vary to some degree in accordance with the psychological situation in which the persons concerned are involved. But the mode of communication is essentially governed by the same archetypal patterns that are at work in artistic communication. Transference phenomena in psycho-analytical practice are also manifestations of archetypal communication. They are synchronous experiences between two psychic systems. The psi-function of telepathic communication seems to be a vital aspect of this archetypal mode of communication.

From what we have so far said, it is clear that the archetypes are collective, in the sense that they are common to all men. Analytical Psychology asserts that the propensity to use archetypal modes is innate in human beings. It believes that the archetypes are inherited in much the same way as the instincts. Man's image-forming proclivity is a manifestation of his archetypal heritage. It is the power of imaging that is inherited, and not necessarily the symbols employed, though the widespread use and acceptance of particular symbols shows that they too are generally recognized as adequate expressions of archetypal experiences.

We must now go on to consider another and vitally important question—that of archetypal motivation in social and political thought and institutions. For it is very necessary for us to understand how archetypal motifs may inform political thinking and find concrete expression in social institutions. Institutions, after all, are made by men; and much may depend

8

on our awareness of the psychological soil in which they are rooted. Take political power and its institutional organization. Political authority is necessarily and of its very nature social. It operates in a multi-lateral system of mutual relationships which distributes appropriate rôles to all the members of society, from the least to the most powerful. What happens if we replace 'social' by 'personal'? The answer is Hitler's Germany or Stalin's Russia. The clue is already given by these phrases, which equate a country with a person. The effect is that the emotions bound up with archetypal authority are now focussed on an individual, who thereby—since the archetype is indestructible—is placed beyond removal and even beyond criticism; his word is the law. Where the archetypal background of political authority is seen, not as social, but in a personalized way, love and justice are the first casualties.

This is what happens under personal dictatorships. But there are totalitarian systems without personal dictators: what is it that makes them so widely acceptable today? We can discern one important reason in the depersonalized character of almost all modern societies: that is, their tendency (mentioned earlier) to press the individual into a specialized mould, so that he lives as a 'part-man' and is cut off from a full experience of personality. Under these conditions man's need to transform himself through unitary experience may well be projected on to the symbols of a totalitarian political system. Putting this another way, we may say that the psychological drive behind contemporary totalitarianism is man's unconscious but frustrated desire to experience himself as a full person. What happens in the political climate of totalitarianism is that the Self, or rather a caricatured form of it, is projected on to a powerful person. This human symbol, the 'Leader' or 'Dictator', by virtue of our projection upon him, has power over us. All this can happen only because we ourselves are 'off-centre'.

It is, I think, of crucial importance to realize that the impulse to project the individual Self on to a social symbol is inspired by unconscious archetypal forces. Only if free societies achieve awareness and understanding of this fact will they be able to find the answer to political totalitarianism whether of the Right or Left. The citizen of a totalitarian society does not distinguish his own individuality from the collective symbol, and so allows the state to become in the end the only arbiter of moral values. The Leviathan, the all-demanding State, is incompatible with the fulfilment of personality. As long as man is regarded as merely a product of society, he is thereby reduced to the level of the primitive. He cannot co-operate with, because he is contained within, his environment. In this respect his thinking is pre-logical. His undifferentiated consciousness, his lack of relationship to personality, reflects his lack of relationship to the organs of government of his society. He is submerged in his political system by reason of the projection of his unitary Self on to his society. The symbolism of the totalitarian State derives its compelling power from the fact that it represents an exteriorization of the archetype Self in a distorted form.

The evolution of consciousness and the becoming aware of relationship to the archetypes are closely bound up with man's search for freedom. This is inevitably so because freedom is the ultimate ethical expression of our deep-seated urge to grow towards full personality. Individual freedom, psychologically understood, is a function of the fully matured personality. This is not to say that man, by becoming consciously aware of them, can cut himself off from his archetypal roots. They will still be there whether he is conscious of them or not. But there is all the difference in the world between the man who is aware of his problem, and the man who is unconsciously ruled by it. The former is, to the extent of his awareness, free; the latter is inevitably bound.

I have left to the end one of the most difficult questions of all. It is whether there is any certain evidence for the existence of the archetypes; and if so, what sort of evidence it may be.

In one sense we can certainly speak of proof; in another sense we can say that it is quite impossible to produce objective proof of the existence of the archetypes. Let me try to explain this with an analogy. In the physical sciences we use concepts such as 'atom' and 'electron' for entities that are not directly observable. There can therefore be no 'proof' of their existence. But the evidence for their existence derives from observation—the observation of phenomena which they serve to explain. To ask 'what' they are is meaningless; for the only way to answer this question would be to describe them in terms of something directly observable and familiar. In fact, they are equated with energy, and energy, as Russell puts it, 'is not defined except as regards its laws and the relation of changes in its distribution to our senses'.[1] In other words we know of something we call energy by inference from observed phenomena; for the same reason we postulate the existence of those complexes of energy which we call atoms and electrons.

Similarly, it is no use asking 'what' the archetypes 'are'; we infer the existence of these 'master patterns' because they are the best way of explaining certain psychic phenomena—the potent, emotionally charged symbolic images which figure in dreams and also in waking mental life. Because we find closely similar images occurring in the dreams and imaginings of many different individuals, often apparently without being related to any experience in the individual's life, we infer that they derive from a heritage of experience, going far back into history, which has been common to some large part of mankind. The empirical interpretation of this common stock of symbolical representations lights up and makes understandable to us our own psychological attitudes and behaviour, and in addition provides us with a criterion of judgment.

All this may seem far removed from the quantitative thinking and experimental methods characteristic of the physical sciences. But should we allow this to worry us unduly? It is true enough that the methodology of the physical sciences is largely inapplicable to the fields either of individual or of social psychology (though even this assertion should not be pushed too far). On the other hand, while the experimental techniques appropriate to the investigation of physical nature have, through their successful application in their own field, come to colour our thinking to a great degree, we should not allow ourselves, because of this, to forget or underestimate the validity of image thinking. With the verbal expression of ideas we are all familiar. With the equally valid use of symbols, much less so. May I illustrate this point with an apposite quotation from Professor H. H. Price. He says: 'If rainbows, reflections, mirages and the like had been less common than

[1]Bertrand Russell, *Knowledge,* p. 256.

they are, philosophers would have denied their existence on *a priori* grounds. For how can there be entities which are at once physical and non-physical, in the physical world and yet not of it, existing from some points of view and not from others, spatial but lacking backs or insides? The fate of mental images in these latter Verbalistic days has been somewhat similar. We have the misfortune to live in the most word-ridden civilization in history where thousands and tens of thousands spend their entire working lives in nothing but the manipulation of words. The whole of our higher education is directed to the encouragement of verbal thinking. Let us hope that our successors will be wiser and encourage both.'[1]

Image thinking is archetypal cognition. It is a mode of experiencing reality in which the mind comprehends as a whole. The revelatory character of a scientific discovery as distinct from its detailed validation, is experienced as a flash of illumination. It is a moment of originality and awe. Doubtless, if the process were analysed, we should find that the whole mental apparatus of memory, sensation and the rest, were involved. Nevertheless, it remains a total response of the personality in which the unitary character of the scientist's mind creatively comprehends a single process. Science advances by bringing ever wider aggregations of data under ever simpler categories. In this process we may see the archetype of unity at work. Since man is potentially a unity and totality in himself, he is inescapably committed to the attempt to experience the world as unity.

We can see the same power at work in the discovery of mental phenomena. In a moment of heightened awareness the discovery of mental inter-relations, unrealized before, has a unique and compelling quality which derives from the fact that the whole of our potentialities of perception are engaged. The whole is more than the sum of its parts. It is that 'plus' which accounts for the compelling, numinous quality which we find in archetypal experience. The unitary character of archetypal apperception conveys in the fullest sense a feeling of truth. It is 'knowing' in the deepest sense; and precisely because it is not and cannot be 'willed', it is an experience of true

[1] *Thinking and Experience* (Hutchinson, University Library), p. 252.

creativity. In this way validation turns into verification; a proof for the experiencing individual as solid as any scientific proof could possibly be. When an individual is brought to find meaning in an otherwise meaningless existence, this is for him 'proof' of the validity of archetypal experience.

Our inquiry into the relationship of man to himself has led us through an intricate maze of philosophical, scientific and mythological thought. If I would try to find the Ariadne's thread to lead us through the uncertainties of human experience, then I would find it in this: that the divine and human processes are expressions of a single theme. This theme is essentially discoverable in those symbols, so full of meaning for us—the archetypes. In following the injunction 'Know Thyself', man is participating in the purpose of creation. For all mankind this purpose is an advance towards fulfilment, towards growth from potential to actual personality.

Let me end with a poem, by F. Pratt Green,[1] which appropriately, and most beautifully, expresses this thought:—

I asked the plum-tree: is there a purpose?
Weighed down by a crop heavy as grief,
It answered, 'the purpose is to be a tree.
What other purpose could there be?'
But I watched it sicken of silver-leaf.

I asked the willow-warbler: is there a purpose?
Young innocent in the thorny brake,
It answered: 'The purpose is to be a bird.
What other purpose could there be?'
But I saw no mercy in the eye of the snake.

I asked my blood-brother: is there a purpose?
Busy at his craft in the sun-washed room,
He answered: 'The purpose is to be a man.
What other purpose could there be?'
When they called him to breakfast he did not come.

I asked the Hidden One: is there a purpose?
Dear and doomed-in brother, bird and tree,
He answered, 'The purpose is creativity.
What other purpose could there be?
Am I not creating you—and you Me?'

---

[1] From *Images of Tomorrow* (S.C.M. Press).

Man as Observer-Predictor

D. M. MACKAY

Lecturer in Physics, King's College, London

'THE SCIENTIFIC and technical world of modern man is the result of his daring enterprise, knowledge without love. Such knowledge is in itself neither good nor bad. Its worth depends on what power it serves. Its ideal has been to remain free of any power.'[1]

I quote these words by the physicist, von Weizsäcker, because I think they set the key for our discussion of the relationship of the scientist with his subject-matter. They emphasize very strongly that the professional relationship of the scientist to his subject matter is a dispassionate, impersonal relationship; and, as you see from my title, I suggest that if we want to give the relationship a name we could call it that of the 'observer-predictor'. By 'predictor', of course, I do not mean 'fortune-teller' but 'calculator'—essentially the observer who wishes to predict by calculations from what he observes—and I use the term to distinguish this relationship from two others.

Very roughly, we can think of three grades of relationship: first, the relationship of *dialogue*, at the level of person with person; then, secondly, there is an observer relationship which is not one of impersonal detachment; it is what you might call the relationship of *observer-participant*. For example, think of a father watching the first steps of his small son. He is an observer, but he is not detached. At the sight of his son's tumbles his

[1] *The History of Nature*, p. 172 (Routledge and Kegan Paul).

15

reaction is not to predict the path which the child's body will take but to leap forward and catch him. He is an observer-participant: he still acts and feels as part of the situation which he is observing. And so both of these can be distinguished from the third relationship of *observer-predictor* in which, as I want to emphasize, the aim of the scientist is to withdraw from the situation as far as possible. He wants to reduce his participation to the minimum. In fact, he wants essentially to answer the question, 'What would the situation be like without me?'

Now this element of withdrawn detachment is necessary for one very good reason, quite a technical one, which has only recently been explicitly worked out. Karl Popper was one of those who recently brought out some of its implications.[1] The point is this, that if you have a predicting, calculating mechanism or human being, such a predicting mechanism cannot possibly predict exactly the future of any system which includes itself. The reason is that if you try to make it allow for the effect of its predictions on the system, it needs to know the prediction before it can calculate what effect this will have, and you simply set it chasing its own tail. It is a point that we will come back to later on in this essay, but I want to emphasize it right at the beginning, because it is the technical reason for the absolute necessity of detachment, of withdrawal from the situation, on the part of the scientist.

Now of course, by saying this I do not mean that the scientist as a man cannot combine other attitudes with that of the observer-predictor. An astronomer who is a religious man may no doubt often be moved to worship, as he looks for the first time on some new galaxy; but when he comes to measure its diameter he measures it in just the same way as anybody else. We do not measure lengths piously; the idea does not make sense.

Nor do I want to deny that in scientific discovery there is a large element of non-deductive, creative thinking which is possible only through an imaginative response by the thinker, and which cannot happen if his attitude is one of complete detachment. To attempt to become completely detached, to become the perfect machine in relation even to scientific

[1]*Brit. J. for Phil. of Science*, vol. I, p. 173.

subject matter, is to become scientifically sterile. One could carry on routine scientific operations quite well, but inventive scientific thinking would become impossible.

My immediate concern is, roughly, with what the scientist is professionally allowed to say about his subject-matter, when he has cleared away the scaffolding of all these other rather logically disreputable operations of imaginative interaction which have enabled him to reach his conclusion. It may be that scientists use the most irrational procedures in thinking up new hypotheses, but when they come to write a paper all this must be cleared away, and the official relationship is that of the dispassionate observer-predictor.

In setting up this relationship of observer-predictor, then, there are two main problems. The first is the problem of withdrawing sufficiently from the situation while still remaining closely enough coupled to it to get information from it. This is, of course, a matter of compromise. The scientist requires something to happen (visibly, or detectably in some other way) in order that he can say anything about the system he is observing; and for something to happen in his observing equipment, energy must pass to it from the system he is observing. So he must interact with the situation; but his problem is to interact with it as little as possible, so as to be able to make a description of what it would have been like if he had not interacted.

The first problem, then, is that of withdrawal, of reducing participation to the minimum. The second problem is the problem of defining a *language*, a connected set of ideas suitable for the detached viewpoint that he has chosen.

I want to illustrate these two problems and the ways in which they are met in two fields where especially interesting features stand out, which I think are relevant to the topic of this symposium. The first field is the study of atomic events—very small-scale events;—and the second is the scientific study of man himself—if you like, meeting oneself as the scientist sees one.

The study of atomic events

Coming first to the study of atomic events, this is a field of very tiny energies, and it is almost a commonplace with us now that in order to extract sufficient energy from such a tiny thing as the atom, in order to be able to say anything about what is happening in it, one disturbs it to an extent which is not negligible. If we are observing a billiard ball, then you might think that in a sense we do not disturb it at all, unless you remember that in order to see it we have to bounce light off it; and bouncing light off something gives it a tiny but definite impact, knocking it in a direction in which it would not have moved if we had not shone light on it. So although a billiard ball, being large enough, takes the impact of the light pretty well in its stride, when we try to observe an atom by shining light or X-rays on it, we may in fact disturb it to an enormous extent, and this results in the famous 'Uncertainty Principle' of Heisenberg. I am not going to stay with that, but you remember his principle: that there is a definite limit to the precision with which we can make predictions about atomic systems, simply because observing a system is deriving information not about the system alone, but about a relationship between the system and you. You observe *interactions*. You do not observe systems by themselves, but interactions between systems and your instruments; and hence statements made about the system by itself are definitely limited in their precision.

So much, then, for the problem of detachment. The second problem is that of defining a suitable language; and this, I think, is a little more interesting from our present standpoint. Right up to the end of the last century scientists had always assumed that there must be one single language-system—one single connected set of ideas—in terms of which everything could be described if only we were clever enough. In the study of light, for example, there was considerable debate between people who thought that the right language to use about light was a language describing it in terms of wave motions, and those who thought that light should be pictured as a stream of particles, and there was a great deal of evidence supporting, oddly enough, both standpoints. But at the turn of the century evidence turned up which led people inevitably to conclude that it was not to be a matter of a *choice* between describing light as wave motion and describing it as particles, but that we had to have *both* languages. In this field one language was not enough; you had to have two complementary languages.

This notion of *complementarity* was a new idea for physics—and for almost everyone else. The idea that it was possible to say that light behaves like waves, which are continuous things, *and* that light behaves like a stream of discrete particles, sounded self-contradictory. And of course it would be a complete contradiction were it not that the situations in which light behaves like waves are different from those in which light behaves like particles. In fact, the language that you have to use is determined by the way in which you have decided to interact with the light. If you interact with the light by making it fall on a detecting instrument—by studying light on *impact*—then it turns out that you have to make your description in terms of particles. If you interact with the light by guiding it in *motion*, then it turns out that you have to use the language of waves, describing the light in terms of waves. The same goes for other entities such as cathode rays, which used to be thought of only as particles. The detailed technicalities are not at all important for our present purpose. I have mentioned them only to illustrate that in science we have discovered that different ways of interacting with a system may lead to quite different descriptions which are not contradictory but complementary, because the situation in which you need to use the one is different from the situation in which you need to use the other.

As a simple sort of analogy of this kind of relationship between two complementary descriptions, you might take the architect's practice of doing plan and elevation drawings of a building. On a plan-drawing you have details which you cannot see on the elevation and on the elevation-drawing you have details you cannot see on the plan-drawing, for the simple reason that each is drawn from a different standpoint. In order to comprehend the whole you have to do a kind of mental synthesis of what it would look like from both standpoints at once. Somehow or other we are able to do this pretty well, even though in fact, if we looked at the real thing, we could see only one view or another according to our standpoint.

So to summarize this example from the field of physics: in studying atomic events we find first that total withdrawal is impossible, that in fact we have to be content with a definitely limited amount of predictability; and, secondly, that, because there are fundamentally two different methods of interacting with an atomic system, we must use two languages and not merely one to describe the system. We will come across similar points now in connexion with our second and main subject, the scientific study of man.

The scientific study of man

In the case of the atom, you remember, the trouble was that the system was so small that the least disturbance we could give to it in observing it knocked it appreciably out of course. Now man of course is a large animal, a good deal larger than a billiard ball, and certainly we do not expect the same kind of unpredictability to apply in the case of man as applies in the case of the atom. In fact, I would like to say in passing that I think we ought to beware of stressing the implications of Heisenberg's uncertainty principle in the case of human beings; above all I do not think it provides the true answer to the old problem of free will and determinism.

But the trouble with man as a scientific subject is that he is himself, of course, an observer: that the system being observed is itself an observer. The scientist studying man, then, is dealing with a sensitive system, in the sense of a system which *amplifies* the effects of his observations. However little you disturb a man by observing him, if the man knows that he is being observed this may have a large-scale effect, so that the man magnifies the effect of your disturbance on him. In engineering jargon, there is 'feedback' in the situation.

A typical example of this, well known to industrial psychologists, arises in what is called time-and-motion study. People thought it would be a very good idea if psychologists could study men at work in a factory, observe how fast they moved, how long it took them to do certain things and so forth, so that in the interests of efficiency one could design the factory accordingly. It soon became known that this was going on; and of course in a very large number of such cases the reliability of the results dropped sharply as soon as the men knew what was happening. A man naturally argues, 'If I work at top speed today, then I shall be expected to work at top speed every day, so I had better go a little more slowly than I normally do'. That is the kind of thing I mean. By observing human beings you may cause disturbances in them on a large scale, no matter how little you are interacting with them; and hence any predictions that you would like to make as a scientist are liable to be invalidated as a result of this interaction.

There is a second difficulty in achieving withdrawal—the scientific prerequisite for prediction—in the study of human systems, namely that if your prediction becomes known it can invalidate itself. This is of course the same logical point with which we started, that a predictor cannot predict the future of a system which includes itself. If, for example, you apply high-powered statistical methods to the Stock Exchange with a view to investing optimally, your prediction might perhaps be valid as long as you do not invest. But directly you allow your decisions to be influenced by your prediction you are in danger of invalidating the basis on which you have made the prediction; and this is quite fundamentally inevitable, because no matter how you try to revise your prediction to allow for the effect of your influence on the system, as soon as you act upon the basis of the revised prediction, you begin invalidating the basis; it is an endless regression.

The same thing happens, of course, in social studies and political studies. For example, you remember the Presidential election in the United States, when one candidate was forecast by the Gallup Poll to be coming in, and in fact the other man was elected. Many people who objected to Gallup Polls said, 'Aha, this just shows how inaccurate a thing a Gallup Poll is.' The moral, however, might well be something quite different. The moral might be that the Gallup Poll was all too accurate, but that in any such case, by publishing your results you automatically modify the system so as to invalidate any prediction based on them. It may be (in many systems it is so), that the *more* accurate your prediction, the more devastating will be its effect on the basis of prediction if you allow it to affect the system.

So in any such situations, if your aim in making a prediction is to act upon the system on the basis of the prediction, there is a very severe limit on the reliability of your action.

This kind of observer-predictor relationship with man-in-the-mass is not quite as politically powerful a relationship as it might seem. One might perhaps, with the help of science-fiction, have thought at one time that the advent of high-speed computors could in principle enable our governors to predict all that we were going to do in such a way that our society would become a perfectly controlled machine with no free will of its own. Since, however, the only purpose of governors in predicting would be to act on the basis of their predictions, in doing so they would certainly restore to us the freedom to falsify their predictions in any respect in which our *physical* liberty was not restrained.

The problem of choice of language

But I think it is under the second heading that we shall find some of the most interesting limitations of the relationship of the observer-predictor in the study of man, namely in the problem of choice of language.

It is a commonplace, of course, that my experience is best and most simply described, to me anyway, in subjective terms; but, of course, these are terms which the observer-predictor is precluded from using. By his terms of reference he must use terms defined from a detached standpoint. He has, in fact, to deal with signs or symptoms of subjective impressions, as observed from outside. Now in choosing a language from an observer standpoint to describe a human being, there are many levels open to us. For instance, if I want to describe what happens as I meet a friend, I might say: 'As I open the door, a mass of pink protoplasm rises to the height of five and a half feet and begins to pucker and wobble up and down noisily'; or I might say, 'He rises to his feet, smiles and greets me heartily', or I might give all sorts of description in between. The bio-chemist could give one in one language, the atomic physicist in another and the psychologist in yet another. There are, then, different levels of language at which we can choose to make the observer-description.

My own work happens to be concerned with trying to describe what goes on in the brain in physical terms, and to focus our ideas we might take a typical problem of the sort I am concerned with: suppose that I decide to move my finger, what is it that goes on at the same time in my head? For many years it was generally agreed, both among those who took the Christian or religious view of the nature of man and those who did not, that if there were anything in the doctrine of the mind or the soul, one ought to come up against some evidence of it (when one tried to push the physical description far enough) in the form of a *gap* in the physical chain of cause and effect. In other words, both those who were in favour of the traditional doctrine of man and those who were against it in the name of so-called materialism, were agreed that evidence for the mind should be expected or sought in some kind of breakdown of physical method at some point in the physical description of the brain and nervous system.

So the need for another language, it was believed, could be shown by trying to push the one language to its limits; you would come across gaps, breakdowns, failures, into which you had to bring something of the other language in order to close the gaps. For example, in the case of my decision to move my finger, the argument was, on the one side, that if you could trace the chain of cause and effect back into the brain you would find some sort of gap into which my decision came; and, on the other side, that if you did not find any gaps, then of course my decision was a 'mere figment' and the 'real thing' was the physical description which was complete. Now I think this is a fallacy, and I believe it arises from a mistaken view of the relationship between the two languages in question—the physical language and, if you like, the mental language—the language in terms of decision, choice, responsibility and so forth.

Complementary descriptions of human activity

What I want to suggest and to work out a little is that these two languages are not rivals but that, like the wave and particle descriptions of light (though not in the same way), they are complementary. I want to stress that they are not complementary in the way in which waves and particles or plan and elevation drawings are, because in these pairs of descriptions both are conceptually on the same level. There is not much difference between the conceptual level of a plan and an elevation drawing. The difference is one of standpoint only. I think a better idea of the relation of the two languages can be got by considering one of those electric advertising signs, made up of a large number of electric lamps on a board forming the outline of an advertisement—say 'Blotto does you Good'. If you were to ask an electrician what was on the board, he could give you a complete description of what was there in terms of electric lamps and wires—a description so complete that you could make a perfect replica of this sign anywhere in the world. Undoubtedly he has left nothing out; but he has not mentioned the 'advertisement' or any of the words in it. On the other hand of course, it would be rather foolish to start an argument with him as to whether he had left something out, because the relationship of the one language to the other is one of complementarity; one is complementary to the other. You find the advertisement not through discovering a fault or a gap in the electrician's self-sufficient description, but by starting all over again with a different attitude to the same data—with a readiness to *read* the sign.

Roughly, the point I want to stress is that the terms in which a question is posed determine the language in which an answer can be sought. If we want to know why lamp number 57 is out, then by asking the question in those terms we invite an answer in electrical language. Conversely, if somebody is ill-advised enough to put up an erroneous statement in electric lamps, it is no good accusing the electrician of incompetence. It is not an electrical defect. The question—what is wrong with this advertisement?—is not answered in electrical terms.

These are of course trivial illustrations, but they bring out the first point, which I think will bear a lot of further exploration: the terms or the language in which you frame your question define for you the terms or the language in which you should properly expect an answer. The reason is simply that any answer which you could attempt to give in the wrong language would already be the answer to a different question—a question phrased in that language. Suppose, for example, we came across the answer, 'Because the wire is cut to lamp 57'. This is an answer to questions of the form, 'Why doesn't lamp

57 light?' You cannot use it alone as an answer to a question of the form, 'Why is this advertisement false?'. On the other hand, one reason why the advertisement offers a better analogy than the others is that there are some ways in which, in practice, we often do sum up both descriptions in one sentence. For instance, we might say, 'I am going to switch on the advertisement', when we mean we are going to switch on the electric current to the lamps. In just the same way, when we speak about man we very often do not mean only one description or the other; we very often mean both, in a rather loose way.

This brings me to a second point: in order that any statement about the system should be true in the one language, it is necessary for some statement to be true in the other. In order that I should say anything at all in advertising language about what is on the board (assuming that I can see it only when it is lit), it is necessary for some electrical statement to be true about what is on the board. Something must be true about the path of electric currents, in order that something describing words delineated on the board may be true. And yet this necessity is not, I think, properly described as a relationship of *causality*. This is perhaps the point I want to emphasize most: that you can have relationships of *necessity* which are not relationships of *causality* in the ordinarily accepted sense of the word. To take an example, where the term 'cause' comes in more naturally: if I write $2x + 3 = 5$ on the blackboard, then in order that any statement, true or false, should be on the board, it is necessary that there should be chalk on the board and that some description in terms of chalk particles be true. But $2x + 3$ is not equal to 5 *because* the chalk particles are in position. It is a relationship of necessity, of complementarity, but not of causality; it is nonsense to speak of one fact as the 'cause' of the other.

Now this has direct bearing on the typical question with which I started. When I decide to move my finger, how is my decision related to what goes on in my brain? Very briefly, I suggest that terms such as decision, choice and so on are words defined from my standpoint as agent or 'actor' in the situation; they form a language of their own, and if I ask what was the cause of my decision to move my finger, the primary answer must be in the same language. It is no good trying to say that the cause of my decision was electro-chemical events in my brain. The reason is that any answer in terms of electro-chemical events in my brain is already the answer to a different question, namely, 'What was the cause of the physical movement which you observed?' You can put it in this way: physiology enables us, in principle we may hope, to trace the pattern of cause and effect right back from the finger movement to the electrical impulses in nerve fibres, to somewhere where it gets lost in the scurry of activity inside the head. No one has begun to trace out the full pattern here, but there has been no evidence so far that normal physical entailment fails. Consequently, we could translate our original question by asking, 'What is the relationship between my decision and the physical events in my head which give rise to the movement of my finger—the physical correlate of my decision?' It is here, I suggest, that the relationship is one of necessity and complementarity, but not causality. In other words, my decision is related to the physico-chemical events in my brain not as cause and effect, but in the kind of way that the description in advertising language is related to the description in electrical language. The one is necessary in order that the other should come about, but it is linguistic nonsense to try to say that one is the cause of the other in the sense in which one would say that the pressing of a button is the cause of the ringing of an electric bell.

There is not space here to discuss the bearing of this on the ancient problem of free will and determinism, beyond suggesting that if we take the typical questions which have been posed in relation to free will and physical determinism and sift them for language systems, asking to what language system each term belongs, I think we shall find a good many instances of mixing of terms from different language systems in the posing of these traditional questions.

Now I do not suppose that many of us here have ever felt very seriously that a complete physical description of man would 'debunk' man. But there are, I suppose, those who do, and I hope it may be clear from this discussion where the fallacy in such debunking lies. Debunking or, as I like to call it, 'nothingbuttery' (the doctrine that man is 'nothing but' a pattern of chemicals, etc.), arises, I think, from the logical fallacy of confusing *exclusiveness* with *exhaustiveness*. To come back to the illustration of the advertising sign, the electrician's account can properly be described as *exhaustive*. It has left nothing out; there is nothing left if he takes away everything on the board according to his description. On the other hand, it is not in any sense *exclusive*. Your description of what is on the board in the words of the advertisement is just as valid at the end of his exhaustive description as it was before, and you do not improve his description by adding at the end of it, 'Oh, and there's also an advertisement saying, "Blotto does you Good"'. It does not belong there.

And so, equally, I think, the physicist has grounds for hoping that in principle (not in practice, because you disturb the system far too much, but in principle) a physical description of the processes of the brain could be complete—exhaustive—in the sense that there would be no gaps into which you would have to fit non-physical processes. But although exhaustive in this sense, it would be in no way exclusive of the description which we would normally give in subjective terms of our own decisions, choices and responsibility.

Perhaps I might add one final remark. As a Christian I have found this case of the scientific study of man, and the relationship between the physical description of man and the mental description, a most helpful and stimulating parable of the age-old mystery of the relationship between the activity of God and the physical events which the scientist studies. I do not mean to suggest in any sense the Pantheistic conclusion that God is just the world we know viewed from a different standpoint; but it seems to me that if one does take the various hints which the Bible and other Christian writings offer as to the relationship of God with the world, it bears much more this stamp of complementarity than of any simple push-button causality. To take just one example, the psalmist speaks of God 'sending His rain upon the mountains' and so on; and he speaks in these terms about so many events for which even he must have known an alternative account in more physical terms, that we would obviously be missing the point if we took his words as an alternative (rival) explanation of the physical cause of the rain. He is using a language complementary with whatever scientific description we can give; and in fact I think that the relationship between most of the religious descriptions of God's activity and what a scientist might have said had he been present, are at least permissively of this logical sort. That is to say, I think it may be worth while exploring the *possibility* that in each case the 'activity of God' is related to the activity observed by human beings, not causally, but complementarily in this sense.

May I summarize in conclusion the two points which I think most important. First, that scientific observation alone cannot give any man the power over his fellows which he has over a machine, as long as he wishes to exercise that power (which is, of course, what we mean by having power)—that in fact the withdrawal necessary for the complete prediction of a system precludes you from interacting with it and using the knowledge that you gain. Secondly, that in any one scientific description of man, as of other systems, we commit ourselves to a choice of standpoint and of abstractive level which is only one among many, and that the validity of descriptions in different language systems must be judged within each language system itself and cannot safely be judged by reference to any description in another language system. This does not mean that the two are totally independent (something must be true in the one language in order that something may be true in the other, and we have come across relationships of necessity between statements in the one language and statements in the other); but the proper criteria of their truth and falsehood are expressed, and can only be applied, in terms of their own language systems. In particular, the validity of any questions of decision, choice and responsibility can be judged, and these questions can be properly answered, only in the language systems of decision, choice and responsibility.

Science and Poetic Insight

MARTIN JOHNSON

Lecturer in Physics, University of Birmingham

Introduction

MANY CONTRIBUTORS to recent discussions of education or
citizenship have expressed dismay at discovering that an abun-
dance of specialized knowledge can entail a shortage of wisdom.
The warning that knowledge without wisdom may be fatal
to civilization does not come solely from those who feel
suspicious about technology; for literary subjects may quite
as justly be suspected of fostering a crudity which is expert but
uncivilized. It is conceivable that the degeneracy occurs in
either type of study when the business of accumulating factual
knowledge becomes an exclusive aim; this aim may ignore or
even supress the growth of discrimination for judging shrewdly
among the possible inferences concerning natural phenomena,
or for appreciating lovingly the achievements of past and
present humanity.

Some of the damage might begin to be repaired by any
determined effort to philosophize over the relations which
connect the two underlying types of mind, uncovering the
differences and likenesses between the scientific attitude and the
imaginative, artistic or poetic, and mystical.

The scientific attitude

Consider, as a tentative basis for discussion, the suggestion
that the essence of all science can be regarded as the arranging

of common experience into an order or pattern which is provisional and never final. Since poetry may also present a pattern from experience, the definition is worth pursuing.

The scientific pattern may be a network of ideas mathematically expressed, as in the physical sciences, or it may be a set of descriptive logical classifications, as in the biological, mental, and social sciences. All sciences like to call their patterns sequences of cause and effect, but the precise meaning of that term can be queried. In every case the 'advance' of science, which is the superseding of pattern by pattern, occurs by bringing an ever wider range of facts under ever simpler categories. The proviso, that the experience be 'common' experience, means that features individual or personal, or determined by local or transient circumstance, are to be eliminated, and the pattern is to emerge as expressing only what is repeatable by successive observers and can be communicated by each observer to the other.

This eliminating of the personal creates the picture of an external 'Nature' independent of its separate observers: this picture may or may not be ultimately an illusion. Thus the most general correlations of facts, laid bare as uniformities expressible in mathematical equations, are usually called Laws of Nature. 'Nature' then becomes the abstraction from every man's experience, the sum total of all facts observed; so the word 'supernatural' drops out of the scientific dictionary as self-contradictory. It could only denote an observing of what is not observable. To retain the word to denote what we do not yet *understand* is an artificiality which pleases some people: but we have little enough understanding of any ultimate substratum which may underlie observable Nature, and no modern scientist pretends to know what Nature is, apart from this restricted meaning of observed fact.

It is clear that this self-discipline of science must be radically separated from the self-disciplines of the arts, because it makes personal emotional preference irrelevant. We do not accept or reject a numerical estimate of the electric charge of an atomic particle because it would be pleasing or unpleasing to 'believe', or because a mystic revelation has uncovered it to some authority, but because repeated impersonal experimenting enforces the high probability of its accuracy until better experimenting may amend it. So the probability of truthfulness grows with the variety of the experiments or observations which yield concordant figures; any law of Nature exemplified in a set of equations attains its slow arduous progress towards a provisional degree of 'scientific truth' the wider the range of verifiable facts that can be expressed in those equations. That is why the sign of advance in science is the dissolving of complex categories into ever simpler and fewer distinct notions, such as, for example, the interaction of electric fields.

An instance of some of these features is the mathematical physics of wave-motion, the kind of phenomenon of which obvious cases occur when water is disturbed or a stretched string is plucked; the law of vibrations and waves gains its generality when we find that light, X-rays, radio, and heat radiation can be shown to obey the wave-equation, as these phenomena exemplify the vibration of electrical and magnetic quantities. The more recent discovery that the behaviour of electrons can also be formulated in the wave-equation is a further gain in unifying our pattern of the external world, since facts so widely scattered as to appear in medical chemistry, in astronomy, in electrical engineering, and in the study of the earth's interior or the earth's upper atmosphere, are all instances of the behaviour of electrons.

But this describing of the electrons themselves by wave-equations introduces also a feature which gives to recent physics considerable novelty in its approach to the meaning of 'knowledge'. If concepts which previously were exclusive to the world of matter, such as the concept of the electron, have become examples of the wave-equation which had also described the world of radiation in empty space, the notion of 'material' has lost the meanings given to it by the science of half a century ago, and has come to share the most characteristic property of the immaterial. So our regard for 'substance' has been replaced by a regard for 'symbol', and we utilize a symbolic wave-equation for calculating an experimentally verifiable fact without hoping or even desiring to picture a 'thing' vibrating in the wave. We seek a pattern, and we no longer ask what it is pattern of or what it is pattern in. We are content to manipulate a mathematical structure if it yields observable fact, but remain happily agnostic about the ultimate nature of whatever exhibits that form or structure. One could be just as good a physicist without 'believing in' the existence of a material world at all, certainly without supposing that nothing but a material world exists—a fancy dear to our scientific ancestors.

Memory and imagination

But if the 'real' in any philosophy of physical science is no longer identifiable with the 'material', we suggest that it may more nearly denote the 'temporal'. Radiation and matter are no longer explained as if they were small-scale or fine-grain models or copies of the large-scale objects of our perception. But because a space-time frame or pattern is still our mode of expressing the resulting experiences, we cannot evade the fact that if *matter* has lost its primitive significance, *time* has not. Science is not interested in a static universe but in the changes which give rise to observation; changes periodic such as reproduction of life or circulation of planets or crystal growth, or changes catastrophic such as the disruption of an atom or of a great star, or changes gradual and statistical such as those we call evolutionary. In all these, the one quantity inescapable which cannot be transformed away is the 'passage of time'; so the fundamental equations of physical science, from the epoch of Newton or of Maxwell, or of today's wave-mechanics of the atom, are all equations denoting variation of some property with time. This is because the scientific account is always a pattern based on the observer's experience, and the most inescapable feature of Nature is that we experience only events in a serial order—a more rational way of stating what common language had called the 'passage of time'.

This unavoidable intrusion of Time emphasizes that science as the arranging of some pattern from experience is always based upon 'sense-data'. For its raw material is always supplied by sight, hearing, touch, etc., and by these senses we detect only alterations in our surroundings, not permanencies. This is still as true today, when unaided senses are reinforced by telescope, microscope, photographic or spectrographic plate, loudspeaker, electrical meters and chronographs and oscillographs.

But the stage from impact of the world upon a human sense, or upon a human-made instrument, to recognition of what the sensation of sight or sound implies, introduces the unsolved problem of perception. Perception, as involving the recognition of what we suppose can cause those sensations, is impossible except for an intelligence based on memory, and also on imagination or the power of creating a coherent mental vision. Take a crude instance of this; while a coin is being looked at from different angles our sight is presented with a succession of differing elliptic shapes. Without memory and some power of imagination, the several shapes would never synthesize into our recognition that there is only one external object, the single circular coin whose appearance from different angles is giving rise to the successive sensations of ellipses.

The physicist's translation of a sensation—for example, the sight of a mark on a photographic plate—into a decision that the path of an electron in a magnetic field denotes a given amount of energy, involves in principle no more mysterious a chain of mental processes than that which underlies the apparent miracle of recognizing the coin, or of recognizing a neighbour's face. The scientist's calculation of an atomic property, and his friend's daily recognition of a commonplace salutation, are both examples, in very differing complexity, of the way the mind builds concepts out of sense-data, imagery, and memory. They differ mainly in that the scientific concepts, such as 'electromagnetic field', 'electric charge', etc., are simple and of verifiable meaning, and therefore have to be free from the impress of the observer's complex individuality which would colour everything by feeling and personality.

This very brief analysis of the relations between Sensation, Perception and Concept, may serve to illustrate our first statement that scientific knowledge is the making of pattern out of common or impersonal experience. This result must dominate the comparison of poetic with scientific attitude. The same analysis has also reinforced our statement that sense-data, underlying scientific as well as everyday experience, are the impermanencies or the changing features in our relationship to any external 'Nature': we could express this by saying that we detect only that which has a time-flux. It is notable that Time has always been a major preoccupation of poets, but with a difference.

Conservatism and progress, poetic and scientific

The features which we have ascribed to the scientific attitude at once confront an opposite in poetry or any of the arts; but the opposition is between ways of pursuing the aim of pattern-building out of experience which is common to science and poetry.

We found that science progresses by eliminating the personal, and reducing phenomena to ever fewer and simpler categories, whereas poetry is mainly concerned with those personal reactions which differ for every individual but recur from age to age. This may perhaps be seen in three characteristics which I have therefore selected for illustration in well-known examples. I shall group the first poems as suggesting how this replacement of scientific unity by aesthetic diversity leads to an interest in irresoluble antitheses, or in situations of conflicting emotion, and therefore to irony as a major poetic theme; the second set are grouped as showing that certain perennial themes underlie the diversity of ancient and modern poetic techniques; the last group show exploitation of the notion of Time, recalling the temporal basis that we ascribed to science. But in these poems Time has the significance of individual feeling instead of denoting the scale for measuring external Nature.

(i) The Greek concept of *eironeia*, inadequately translated as 'irony', can express the poetic preoccupation with the opposition between incompatibles, such as for instance fulfil-ment and frustration. The following might be compared, for illustration: Donne's 'Go and catch a falling star', whose material is of the simplest fantasy; Shakespeare's sonnet 'Fare-well, thou art too dear for my possessing', which employs a more complex and subtle imagery; two modern pieces of realism, Housman's ''Tis time, I think, by Wenlock Town', and Dylan Thomas' 'The hand that signed the paper felled a city'. None surpass in force the extreme simplicity of expression in the Homeric lines where Odysseus returning in disguise is

34

recognized only by his aged dog: 'But upon the dog Argos came the blackness of death in the moment of recognition in the twentieth year of absence'. A nearly Homeric simplicity in recent times is regained in the first and last stanzas of Hopkins' 'Felix Randal'.

(ii) Scientific impermanence, the incessant supersession of old by new, finds opposing counterpart in the perennial recurrence of a few poetic motifs under the fluctuating technique of extremely different ages. This may be illustrated by comparing Vergil's vision of the shades pressing in frustration to cross the river of death, with Shakespeare's King Lear awakening to half-recognition of Cordelia, and with Wilfrid Owen's 'Red lips are not so red as the stained stones kissed by the English dead'. Seldom has writing so supremely expressed the situation of desperate pity, and the unforgettable element in our personal response is identical over the twenty centuries.

Another poetic preoccupation, that of terror, may similarly be discovered as perennial under subtly differing techniques, by reading first Dante's approach to the infernal city of Dis, then de la Mare's dream of awakening to the death of the beloved, 'Who now put dreams into thy slumbering mind?' For the very different theme of tranquillity, I suggest reading Dante's emergence into the Earthly Paradise, Spenser's *Prothalamiom* with its soporific refrain, 'Sweete Themmes! runne softly, till I end my Song', and de la Mare's aged shepherd, 'His are the quiet steeps of dreamland, the waters of No More Pain'.

All these moods have a permanence unlike the essential fluidity and progressiveness of scientific history; indeed a prototype of all that has been quoted, and in no wise inferior, might be found in the Homeric dialogue of Hector and Andromache over their child on the eve of the destruction of Troy.

(iii) I claimed that Time is the essential feature of quantitative science, but scientific time is definable in terms of scale-measure, whereas for poetry the whole concept is coloured by the human reaction to opportunity and the irrevocable. There is perhaps no briefer and more devastating epitome than Housman's 'Tarry delight, so seldom met, so sure to perish'. The theme is familiar classically in Shakespeare's sonnets, for example those beginning, 'When I do count the clock that tells the time, and see the brave day sunk in hideous night', and 'When I consider every thing that grows holds in perfection but a little moment'. In place of the resentment of the Elizabethan might be quoted Keats' ecstatic acceptance of Time in his first lines of 'Endymion'; it is perhaps unexpected that in the present age the poetry of the acceptance of Time reappears in the last stanzas of C. Day Lewis' 'Sky wide an estuary'. A more contemplative vision of the significance of Time has never been better expressed than in de la Mare's 'Very old are the woods'. For subtle imagery, Eliot's encounter with the spirit of the dead in 'Little Gidding' is as poignant as anything said by the older poets, and many readers will return also to Wilfrid Owen's 'Strange Meeting'. Eliot's preoccupation with Time differs from that of the Elizabethan and Victorian minds in expressing, not the common resentment, but realization that Time is supreme mystery, and that to love a mystery unsolved is a step towards wisdom.

Technique and mere technique in poetry and science

We have stressed the contrast between poetic evocation of varied individual imagery and the essential singleness of meaning in a scientific concept. This situation carries with it a contrast in technique. The imagery which crystallizes experience into a scientific concept or scientific law must be compounded out of the quantitative features accessible to all other explorers in similar experimenting; whereas for the poetic image, any fantasy will be legitimate if it proves powerful in evoking individual states of feeling, according to infinitely varied memories. Therefore what would be pernicious nonsense in law, history, or science, may be divine nonsense in poetry, and not necessarily delusive at that. Homer and Vergil are not 'out of date' by clothing their immortal human sympathy in the imagery of souls which descend with the sun into the west, or of the dead who cross their dark river.

The danger at once arises that a poet may become obsessed by mere technique, and the glory of mystery degenerate into obscurity or mystification, which is abhorrent alike to science and to any art. Scientists more readily restrain one another from this danger, but their own corresponding temptation is to let the terms of their employment drown them in mere gadgetry and a forgetfulness of the aim to see Nature as comprehensive pattern.

I would suggest a study of the following poems as indicating ways by which mere technical skill develops into technique as legitimate means for arousing a state of mind. Begin from Yeats' 'Byzantium', Swinburne's 'Alas but though my flying song . . .' from the elegy on Beaudelaire, the 'Psyche', of José-Maria de Heredia, and the 'Apparition' of Mallarmé. The subtle stage at which, without demanding explicit restriction to 'meaning', a piece of verbal music develops power to convey a coherent mental imagery might be illustrated by the following poems; Shelley's 'Night'; Meredith's 'Lovely are the curves of the white owl sweeping,' from *Love in a Valley*; de la Mare's 'Sweep thy faint strings, musician'; and more recently Stephen Spender's 'I think continually of those', where a finale of verbal music contributes powerfully to the vision of the past: 'Born of the sun they travelled a short while towards the sun, and left the vivid air signed with their honour'.

We end with a query: can legitimate technique include dissection and reassembly of a language? In many cases this is a mere refuge of those whose command of normal usage is inadequate to their task, and recent arts are littered with such; but it is impossible to dismiss Hopkins in those terms. Three sonnets may be quoted, 'Carrion Comfort', 'Caged Skylark', 'No worst, there is none', as conveying an impression as sharply cut as any in more conventional writing. There is also the dissection and seemingly random re-assembly of the poetic image itself; here it is not so easy to acquit Rilke of wanton obscurity, for example in the third of the *Sonnets to Orpheus*, 'Gesang ist Dasein. Für den Gott ein Leichtes. Wann aber sind wir?' Obscurity of image is more readily detected and arrested in scientific discipline than in the arts. Clarity of image is so great an asset as to be mentioned with honour even when the poetic content is slight; for instance, Masefield's 'Cargoes'.

The border between science, poetry, and mysticism

The contrast between scientific and poetic significance of Time is one example of those disparities between the two ways of making pattern from experience which raise the insoluble query, 'Does either provide insight into reality or truth?' I have written elsewhere about scientific and aesthetic criteria for these impossibly ambiguous words, and here there is space only to draw briefly some distinctions.

While poet and moralist, since Homeric days and earlier, have regarded clear-sightedly the fading of treasured memory and the inevitability of regret over fleeting opportunity, philosophers since Plato until nearly yesterday conceived as an urgent aim the explaining away of this, our destined slavery to Time. Some have even fallaciously invoked Einstein and relativity physics as ally. But to call in physics to redress an adverse balance in spiritual destiny has been a rash hope: we have emphasized that science is essentially a study of time-changes, but to the ultimate nature of Time it can afford no clue. Time in physics is a question of correlating quantitatively one set of events with another set which happens to define a scale. Extrapolated today to the subatomic on the one hand and the cosmic on the other, the differential equations involving time cannot even be formally dissected without limit. In atomic physics we find ourselves unable to adapt the large-scale perceptual treatment of time to the smallest intervals, while even the earliest and least controversial relativity enforces the fact that intervals are not uniquely dissectable into temporal and spatial. In astronomical cosmology it has become as indeterminate to argue about the 'beginning of Time', since an origin of the universe can be transformed in its equations into an infinite regress of permanent existence by altering the time-scale from the direct to the logarithmic, as de Sitter, Milne, Eddington, Dirac, and others have shown, and I have reported in some detail in a recent publication.

But two types of mind have, without any such spurious attempt to borrow from physics, sought to deny the 'reality' of Time; they have thereby contended that the temporal sequence of our individual experience, and also of science's 'common' experience, is some sort of illusion from which escape is possible and desirable. Firstly there are those explicitly acknowledged to be mystics, and secondly those metaphysicians who have chosen to assume that the universe is a multifarious manifestation of a single unity whose nature is not material.

The category of mystic must include the great Chinese visionaries of the ancient Taoist culture, also the Chinese modifiers of Buddhism, and their European counterpart, the great Catholic saints of our monastic centuries. Wisely all these genuine mystics refrained from arguing: they simply stated that they found themselves able to train a sense of unity with Nature which liberates them from Time. Each mystic retains his inalienable right to his inner feeling, but none of them has right to claim conveyance of that state of mind to other minds. The 'unreality' of Time remains for each of them secret, personal, undemonstrable but individually satisfying. The metaphysicians, on the other hand, Plato, Plotinus, Spinoza, down to Bradley and McTaggart of the present century, incorporated into their discourse a persistent claim to prove logically that Time is unreal. Such proofs are always fallacious, since they depend on uncovering self-contradictions in the concept of Time which have yielded to later discoveries in logic.

It is possible that we see in these great idealists, as in Eddington's love for the Kantian notion that Time is the mind's own imposition upon Nature, the curious fact that the acutest logical mind often contains within itself the germ of the mystical. As especially with Spinoza, the philosophy of Time's unreality is actually an expression of the mystic hidden in incongruous logical guise, and lacking only the subtlety which it might have gained from poetic imagery.

We never quite evade the feeling that some personalities are less subject than others to the dominion of Time: man lives not solely upon his sense-knowledge of an external world, and if his organization of his own internal world carries him to sufficient mental stature, he does continually create the more lasting by selecting in memory and imagination from the most transient of delights and terrors.

Now that is exactly what we found that the poet is doing.

But to estimate how lasting an individual's mental or spiritual creation will be, is certainly to dream: it is not a possibility of conscious intellect but of a faith that what we most lovingly construct is never a total loss. Many men have experienced an unprovable but ineradicable and powerful sense that there is a personal response—and perhaps a responsibility—in the universe at large, to which the decays of Nature are not the final word. This may well be the basis of genuine religion, but is wider than any single orthodoxy and will survive many theologies, and it is idle to deny that this instinct has always existed even in our uttermost disasters. But such imaginative spirit ought to claim its subtle validity without asking spurious logical support; for a disciplined imagination is not a contradiction of the logical, but complementary to it, since we showed earlier that without memory and imagination not even the simplest scientific concept could emerge from the flux of sensation.

All those mystical attitudes to Time and the universe serve to exhibit a reaction to experience radically differing from the scientific, and it is inevitable to inquire the status of poetic insight in that company. Poet, artist, and lover share something of the standpoint of the worshipper, who by his sacrifice to the 'practice of an unseen presence' does actually find the material and temporal world well lost, and all four are possibly the only ones among us to realize *aeternitas* within our own time. There is no ground in science or philosophy for denying this reality of a Presence that some will call Divine, the cherishing of which is the true meaning of prayer when one can penetrate thereto through the fog of the conflicting creeds. But if the poet, with the worshipper, are inevitably thus mystics, they must not demand a logical as well as an imaginative or spiritual triumph over the prison of Time which we share with the animals and plants and the inanimate world.

Experience and imagery

The contention that a poetic view of Time could be akin to that of the mystics who include worshipper, lover, and idealist philosopher, will be resented in many quarters. I am, however, using the word mystic to denote not the confusion of thought more justly termed mystification, which we found abhorrent to the techniques of science and poetry alike, but to denote the acceptance of aspects of experience inexpressible in the space-time frame of science.

In fact the one legitimate anchorage by which the situation could be judged lies in experience. When some experience, stabilized with deeply planted memories, is so strong as to overpower a man's acceptance of his fellows' valuation of the good or beautiful, his imaginative cultivation of the experience may reach a stage describable only as worship; ethical and aesthetic terms are no longer adequate, and something has become Sacred to him, calling forth a devotion beyond logical assessment or justification. This sense of 'holiness' is as genuine to the individual as is his notion of an external 'material' world, but it is not always repeatable at will and cannot readily be passed on to other people. It has thus a privacy contrasting vividly with the fact that science does not become knowledge at all until it can be communicated and its data recovered by a repetition in some colleague's measurements.

It has been supposed that because no man can share, still less dictate, the imagery of another man's most intimate experience, that therefore the religious aspect of the mystical in all of us is delusive, an idle dream of wishful thinking. Such supposition seems to me fallacious, and the fallacy is often aggravated by 'rationalists' in stigmatizing the notion of the Divine as an 'unnecessary hypothesis'. The Divine Presence is not a hypothesis or theory for explaining things, but is a fact of direct experience by millions of individuals. We may blame the ecclesiastics who pretend that the mystical is provable as though it were logic, for this error of associating the Divine with a hypothesis. Theology, made for an age when metaphysics was an asset, not a liability, has thereby obscured the status of legitimate imagery, for instance that of the New Testament; in that imagery both learned and unlearned can together discover that all we can know or need to know is through the symbolism of Fatherhood, Brotherhood, or the Communion of the Saints. These pictures, whether regarded as the religious or the poetic prerogative of the mystic in all of us, are instances of the fact that the imaginative is not necessarily the untrue or delusive. They would not gain by logical demonstration: for when we all, from time to time, exercise every man's privilege of being the child crying out in fear of the dark, the Divine answer is there for us, but is not to be held up to public exhibition. Our 'belief' in it is not the mere under-writing of an unintelligible metaphysical creed, and can indeed function without the latter; belief is rather the practice of steering experience in the light of a mystic's symbols re-created in the imaginations of all of us.

On the other hand, the status of the poetic impulse may be the creation of imagery for public expression of that level of experience whose private cherishing contained the essence of worship.

I have been considering religion in a far wider sense than any tied to the churches and their conflicting creeds. So I base this meaning of worship on recognition that something important exists other than the universe of concepts constructed by scientific method out of the sense-data ordered in a space-time frame. To come to terms with this recognition is the private religion of each of us; but a man possessing not only the instincts of creative imagination but also a disciplined sense of craftsmanship will not live solely in the loneliness of individual worship of whatever he discovers sacred, but will seek expression in poetry and the arts of this deepest ecstasy of pity, terror, love, exhaltation or despair.

We all respond to a poem according to the private store of memory and imaginative power, which is different in each of us; this fluctuating reinforcement would be totally irrelevant in science, but it confers upon poetry its glory of enabling today's reader to enter intimately the spiritual adventure of the long-dead writer. The struggle towards scientific truth involves the repeating of the researcher's original measurements to find under what conditions they are substantiated, but the consummation of the poet's creativeness involves the leap of imagination in each appreciating mind in answer to the artist's original stimulus. It is to evoke this multifarious answer that the poet must become supremely sensitive in perception and self-disciplined in technique: he can then enshrine his experience in the exquisite word-pattern capable of unlocking the secret places of the individual memories, delicate, tremendous, or poignant as they severally may be. Let not either poet or scientist despise each the other's exploitation of imagery and memory, and let each have the humility to recognize that a mind busy at the one kind of pattern-making from experience can gain by even a distant glimpse of the disciplined creativeness demanded from the other. It is more possible in poetry than in science to degenerate into the chaos of ignoring the community of minds, so the poet can learn much from the rigorous training undergone by the scientist. But the scientist, treating for the purpose of his technique the world of Nature as if independent of the observer, can equally learn from the poet that the imaginative is not also necessarily the imaginary; for the poet is less liable than the scientist to forget that there is an internal as well as an external world.

Ritual in Society

A. MACBEATH

Professor of Logic & Metaphysics, Queen's University, Belfast

RITUAL IS A DIFFICULT and complex subject for two main reasons. First, it is not one thing but many. We find religious and secular ritual, political and legal ritual, ritual connected with eating, with marriage, with death, and so on. It is therefore doubtful if any significant statement can be made about it which does not admit of many exceptions. For the different forms of ritual are responses to different situations and serve different purposes in the life of the individual and of society. Men engage in ritual activities for different reasons. The activities arise from different impulses, are accompanied by different beliefs, and express or arouse different emotions. Each activity poses the questions—Does it owe its significance (1) to the situation to which it is the response, or (2) to the beliefs or emotions which it expresses or arouses, or (3) to its ritual form, or (4) to all three? The answers may be different in the case of different ritual activities.

Secondly, no piece of ritual is self-contained or self-explanatory. The observable behaviour which we describe as ritual is only one element in a total reaction to a situation, an element which cannot be understood or even exist by itself. For man not only acts but thinks and feels, and action and thought and feeling are closely inter-related in the life of the individual. Similarly in religion, ritual observances, beliefs and dogmas and emotional attitudes are inextricably intertwined, and in the

45

way of life of a society the different aspects, the ideas and purposes, the attitudes and activities, cannot be understood in isolation. Accordingly, whether we consider ritual as an activity of an individual, as a religious phenomenon or as a factor in the life of a society, we cannot tear it from its context and consider it in abstraction without distorting its nature.

The consideration of ritual, therefore, raises fundamental psychological questions about the inter-relation of the different elements of human nature, such as the relative casual priority of emotions, beliefs and impulses to action. It raises similar questions about the inter-relation of the different factors in religion, the emotional attitudes, the ritual practices, and the beliefs and dogmas, and about the interconnexion of the different aspects of the way of life of the society or group concerned.

What are the attitudes which promote the ritual activities and the beliefs which sustain these attitudes? Are the ritual acts sustained at the outset by any beliefs, or are dogmas and myths rationalizations to explain and justify behaviour in which men engage independently of them? Again, what sort of situations occasion ritual activities? What are the purposes of those who engage in them? What emotions find expression in or are aroused by the activities? What psychological and social effects do they produce? Are the situations to which ritual is the response merely the occasions of the ritual activities, while the form which the activities take are determined by other factors, such as social tensions? And so on.

There is, I think, no single or simple answer to such questions. The answers vary from one kind of ritual to another, and perhaps from one individual or one society to another, and some of the questions may not be legitimate at all because they are based on false assumptions about the casual relationships between the factors concerned. We find one anthropologist or historian of religion or writer on ritual putting forward a theory which covers certain forms or certain aspects of ritual and generalizing it as if it applied to all, and another putting forward a different theory that covers other forms or aspects. Such theories, so far as I can see, are not so much opposed or contradictory as supplementary. Each has got hold of a part of the truth but states it as if it were the whole. Thus, one theorist holds that the function of ritual is to give courage and confidence, to strengthen morale, and another that its function is to cause concern and anxiety; one that its function is to meet certain needs of the individual, another that it is to contribute to the survival of society; whereas, in fact, it may well do both and perhaps cannot do the one without also doing the other.

The question which none of these theorists seems to ask is, Why is there ritual at all? What is there in the human mind, what is the psychological element, which is the source of the tendency to run to ritual? All they seem to be concerned with is: What is the particular impulse or the particular need from which, or round which, a specific sort of ritual arises? Yet the universality of ritual and the diverse forms which it takes suggest that there is something in human nature to which it is congenial, some need which it meets, some situations to which it is the natural response.

In dealing with a subject which is so complex and raises such fundamental issues I can touch on only a few points, and what I have to say about them is tentative and provisional. Indeed, I shall be largely concerned with asking questions to many of which I shall not attempt to give an answer, for the simple reason that I am not certain which, if any, of several answers is the correct one, and I doubt if there is any answer which applies equally to all forms of ritual.

I do not propose to begin with a definition of ritual, for two reasons. First, there are so many different forms of ritual that any definition covering them all would not give us much insight into the nature of any, or indicate everything that we normally mean by the term. This is true, for example, of the definition given in the *Oxford Dictionary*. Ritual is there defined as (1) a prescribed order of performing religious or other devotional services, and (2) a custom or practice of a formal kind. This is unexceptionable as far as it goes, but it seems both to cover activities which should not be regarded as ritual in the full sense and to leave out much of what we mean by the term.

My second and more important reason for not attempting a definition is this—Ritual seems to me to occur in more and in less developed forms, and the concept of ritual contains ideal or normative elements which are not fully realized even in the most developed forms. And there are decadent as well as undeveloped forms of ritual. Whether or not we apply the term ritual to the decadent and undeveloped forms is largely a verbal question.

I might illustrate the sort of concept that ritual seems to me to be by reference to the concept of the State or of religion. In these cases the completed concept, what the State or religion is capable of being, what we mean by the terms, can be present in a given case in a greater or a lesser degree, and perhaps it is not completely present in any actual instance. To understand such concepts, perhaps the best way is to analyse their most developed forms and consider how far others approach to these.

What, then, are the elements or factors which enter into the completed concept of ritual—that is, into ritual in the full sense as we find it, for example, in religious or magico-religious ritual? Ritual is something which we do. It has, therefore, an outward and visible form. It is, in fact, the external and therefore the social aspect of religion, or religion in action. As a form of observable outward behaviour, ritual is, or involves, the repetition of precise forms of activity, gestures, words, tones, demeanours. These activities need not be elaborate or splendid; they need not involve pomp or pageantry; they may be simple and severe, but they must be formal and stylized and they must be repeated precisely and accurately.

In this respect, the tendency of the human mind towards ritual activities is one expression of its tendency to form habits. But mere routine or habit, however precisely repeated, does not constitute ritual. For the observable activities in ritual are not self-explanatory; they are symbolic. They have a meaning which is not discoverable merely by empirical observation; a meaning which the individual cannot learn for himself, as he can the purpose of ordinary practical activities. He has to be taught the meaning of ritual, initiated into it. In that sense ritual is conventional. The ritual activities as seen by the external observer may seem trivial or insignificant, and entirely disproportionate to the weight of significance which they convey to the initiated. Their meaning is not intrinsic, but acquired. For this reason they are sometimes said to be routine activities which do not directly promote the physical well-being of the actors. But this account, while true, is apt to be misleading. In considering it, we must distinguish between the point of view of the actors and that of the external observer. For activities which are intended by the actors to promote their physical well-being and which, in fact, do so, may be performed in a ritual manner, and the actors may believe that the ritual manner of performing them is necessary to produce the practical results which follow.

For example, the primitive may believe that tilling the field and sowing the crops in a ritual manner may help the crops to grow, and even in the most developed and rational religion hopes and expectations and appeals for practical results are mingled with the motives of the devout performer as he takes part, for example, in a marriage ceremony, or in a service for rain or for the return of peace; so that the ritual character of the activities consists not so much in the kind of acts performed as in the manner in which they are performed. The manner gives them a significance which they would not otherwise have. Apart from it, they might produce the practical results which the agent intends, but they would not produce the psychological and social effects on him and on his fellows which even the outside observer can see.

These effects are usually referred to by anthropologists as the functions of the ritual. But however important the results of ritual may be, men do not engage in ritual activities in order to produce them. Ritual can produce these results only if the actors consciously and deliberately aim at, or intend, something else. For example, the primitive does not engage in magico-religious ritual in order that he may have courage and confidence, but in order that the rain may fall and the crops grow, and unless he believes that his ritual activities will produce these effects, they will not give him courage and confidence. But whatever be the conscious purpose of the actors in performing ritual activities, and whether or not these have any utilitarian purpose, ritual activities are the outward expression of certain attitudes of mind, especially emotional attitudes. Without these inner attitudes, the mere external observances or activities are not ritual in the full sense. That is why we find the ancient Chinese Record of the Rites beginning, 'Always and in everything let there be reverence.' When the external observances become mechanical and lifeless we have ritual in decay, religion at a low temperature, and ritual can no longer fulfil its functions either in the life of the individual or of society.

Ritual is an expression of the urge to express and to communicate, to give external and visible form to certain experiences and to convey them to others. Its appeal is primarily to the emotions rather than to the intellect, to the heart rather than to the head. It impresses without explaining, it produces results without giving reasons. Indeed, it tends to still the unsettling doubts of critical thought. That is one of the ways in which it gives comfort. It is also one of its dangers, the danger of being regarded as a substitute for, rather than a supplement to, the critical processes of the intellect. In the modern western world, especially among the better educated and more intellectual sections of the community, the main emphasis even in religion tends to be on beliefs, on conceptual thought and clear ideas, on what can be adequately expressed in words. It is therefore more difficult for us to appreciate the full significance of ritual in the lives of other societies, and even in the less intellectual and less reflective sections of the community in every society. Hence we are apt to under-estimate the importance in human life of the non-rational elements and their expression. But man is not merely an intelligence; and the practical and emotional aspects of life which find expression in ritual activities must be allowed to play their part. In a well-integrated personality and a well-ordered society each side of human nature has to be developed and given scope for free exercise. The difficulty is to maintain a proper balance between them; for while the non-rational experiences are needed to supplement the activities of the critical intellect, the emotions and the ritual activities in which they find expression need the continuous criticism of rational thought to keep them within proper bounds.

Why then is ritual necessary to express, to arouse, to intensify, and to communicate certain experiences? Why do we need forms of expression and communication other than verbal?

There are certain psychological attitudes which cannot be directly evoked or communicated. Take emotion, for example. I cannot directly communicate my emotion to another person. I can show, say, my respect for him, only indirectly, by behaving in an appropriate manner. If I want to share my feelings with another, the best way is to engage with him in the sort of activities which are most likely to produce such feelings. Nothing is more conducive to arousing a feeling in a person than to see its appropriate expression in another. I cannot directly, by mere willing or by any other direct means, evoke even in myself a feeling which is not there. If I want to evoke such a feeling, the procedure which is most likely to be successful is to put myself in a certain situation or to behave in certain ways. Moreover, feeling is evanescent and cannot be directly recalled, or it may be weak and need strengthening. Thus, to evoke it in myself or another or to strengthen or to communicate feeling, practical activities, indirect means, are necessary, and in the case of certain feelings these practical activities must be of a ritual kind. Why this must be so we shall consider shortly.

Meantime, I want to note that there are experiences not only of an emotional kind but also of a cognitive or quasi-cognitive kind, thoughts and beliefs and insights, for which we cannot find adequate conceptual expression. We cannot express them clearly or adequately in words, and so we cannot make them clear to ourselves or communicate them directly to others. Such thoughts and experiences we can express and communicate only indirectly, by means of metaphors and symbols and myths—the materials of ritual. In the practice of ritual activities, and in living through the emotional experiences which they arouse, we seem to become aware of a profound significance which we can at best express only partially in words. This is especially true of experiences into which the sense of the supernatural enters—a sense which is not adequately conveyed by clear intellectual concepts but which nevertheless seems to be a form of apprehension.

The analysis of such experiences presents a very difficult psychological problem. We do not seem able to characterize the objects of which we seem to be aware in such experiences except in terms of the experiences, especially the emotional experiences, which they produce in us. Nevertheless, in living through the experiences and the activities which give rise to them we seem to become aware of something which is in danger of being restricted, if not destroyed, by attempts to express it in the rigid concepts of the intellect. To evoke and to communicate such experiences we need ritual activities. Certain forms of ritual are the dramatized expression of certain beliefs and attitudes, and to take part in the ritual tends to evoke the beliefs and attitudes when these are absent and to strengthen them when they are weak. It does this without giving evidence, and at times against the available evidence. That is one of its dangers. It may prevent people from considering the evidence for the dramatized beliefs objectively, and may lead them to accept such beliefs not only when there is no evidence to support them, but also when the available evidence is against them.

But why do such experiences, whether emotional or quasi-cognitive, require for their expression and communication not only practical activities, but ritual? If the experiences themselves and the beliefs associated with them are so vague and varying, why do they require such formal, rigid, precise, unvarying activities for their expression?

There are certain characteristics of ritual which seem to make it appropriate for the expression of the experiences aroused on certain occasions, especially occasions which are regarded as important because they arouse strong emotion and fire the imagination:

(1) Ritual is impersonal. It is not the person so much as the part he plays which is regarded as important. Ritual drops out the purely private and personal. It is a social rather than an individual activity and therefore it is a great equalizer, like a military uniform. In the performance of his ritual rôle, therefore, a person may do things which would be deeply resented if he did them in his individual capacity.

(2) Ritual has a certain dignity, a seriousness and a solemnity. There is a considerable aesthetic element in it which satisfies a certain aspect of our nature. Why its precision and its formal nature should make it appropriate on important occasions, or

as the expression of certain emotions, is difficult to say. We can no more say, for example, why certain patterns of colour or combinations of sound are specially pleasing. All we seem able to say in these cases is that the stuff of which we are made seems to work better in some ways than in others. Which activities are more pleasing or comforting we have just to learn by experience, and perhaps we cannot give any other reason why this should be so. One experience or attitude finds its most adequate expression in poetry, another in clay, another in music, and still another in ritual activities, and what is expressed in one form cannot be completely translated into another. But while this may be true of the ritual form as such, it may still be the case that the content of the ritual, the actual activities in which the people who practice the ritual find comfort, are determined by factors in their own social life, factors which may vary from one society to another. This may partly explain the fact that while we find ritual in all societies, the activities in which it consists vary from time to time and from society to society. This point has been illustrated in detail by Professor Gluckman in his Frazer Lecture on Rituals of Rebellion in South-East Africa.

(3) Ritual can remain the same while the experiences, the beliefs, the attitudes and the emotions which find expression in it or to which it gives rise may vary, sometimes in kind and more often in degree of intensity, from individual to individual and from time to time in the life of the same individual. And (4), there seems to be an inevitability, a feeling of rightness about ritual, a feeling which demands precise and accurate performance.

Ritual resembles language and art in that all three are media both of expression and of communication. Perhaps all of them were at first mainly or even solely expressive, but in the course of their development language has become mainly a medium of communication and art has remained mainly expressive. Ritual performs both functions, but it has closer affinities with art than with language. But ritual tends not only to express, to arouse and to communicate emotion; at times it also restrains and controls it and directs it into certain channels. This is specially important in situations which naturally and normally arouse emotion so intense that it may be in danger of getting out of control. When, for example, a person's friend dies, or his son or daughter is being given in marriage, he is uneasy and restless. He may have a part to play, and in any case he wants to do something to relieve the tension. The socially prescribed ritual indicates the way in which it is appropriate for him to behave and to express his emotions. In the same way the primitive, in the presence of forces which he does not understand and cannot control, such as those of birth and death, storm and drought—forces which arouse in him the sense of the supernatural and about which he feels impelled to do something— finds in ritual the answer to his need. It provides not only an outlet for his emotions but something which consoles and comforts him and gives him courage and confidence in the face of trials and difficulties. Or again, when a meal is taken among people of another class or from another country, a knowledge of the appropriate ritual puts the individual at his ease and overcomes his sense of awkwardness and enables him to express appropriately his respect for his hosts. Similar considerations apply to the conventional ritual of ordinary everyday human relations, in family and professions. It prescribes the appropriate way of expressing respect for others; it restrains undue intrusion on their privacy or undue coldness towards them. It tends to produce, as well as to express, the appropriate emotional attitude towards them.

This brings to light another function which ritual fulfils. In cases where the individual does not feel the appropriate emotions towards others, or fails to appreciate the importance of an occasion, the performance of the prescribed ritual may bring home to him how he ought to feel or how important the occasion is. If he behaves as if he felt, he may come to feel. This is the aspect emphasized by Radcliffe Brown, who holds that ritual produces the very sense of anxious concern that others say its main function is to relieve. Now there is no doubt that, in the case of some individuals and on some occasions, this may be so, but this does not mean that we can found a general theory on it, or that its being so is inconsistent with the theory that the normal effect of ritual is to allay anxiety and ease tension.

For example, it is normal for parents to feel anxious before the birth of a child, but some may not feel any anxiety, and in their case the fact that among their people a certain ritual is prescribed for them on such occasions may itself produce uneasiness—uneasiness that if the ritual is not accurately performed, all will not be well with mother and child: this brings home to them the importance of the occasion and how they ought to feel about it. But however the anxiety is produced, the effect of duly performing the ritual practices is to allay it. And the situations to which ritual is the response are situations which in themselves normally arouse strong emotions. They are situations which for one reason or another are regarded as important, generally because they are believed to affect the well-being or even the life of the individual or his group. They are situations of tension, of crisis, or at least of embarrassment. Such situations are very varied, depending on the knowledge and experience of the people concerned. They may be religious or they may be secular, and one form of ritual may have among one people a religious, and among another a secular, significance. This is true, for example, of the rites of marriage or of coronation. But I suspect that there is in all ritual a mystical element, a sense of mystery, a sort of religious thrill; and those anthropologists may be right who believe that all ritual was in origin religious, or magico-religious, and that other forms of ritual are decayed forms.

It is certainly the religious forms which have had the most important effects in promoting the mental integrity of the individual and the social solidarity of the group. Nothing unites people more closely than the common experience of intense emotion, common concern for common objects, and the more intense the experience which they share in common the more closely it unites them, and no experience is so deeply moving as that in which the sense of the supernatural is present. Hence, religion has always united those who share it and separated them off from others.

Here I am skating over thin ice and trying to evade a fundamental issue which has deeply divided social anthropologists but which I have no space to discuss adequately—Does the sense of the supernatural come first and give rise to the emotional experiences which then find expression in ritual activities, or do the ritual activities come first and give rise to the emotion, and is the sense of the supernatural anything more than a name for the experiences which men have when they act collectively in a ritual way?

Today the prevailing theory among many, if not most, social anthropologists and historians of religion is that the earliest form which religion took among mankind was that of ritual practices, and certainly there has been no religion without rites. According to this view, in the presence of certain situations which concern the vital interests of the group, situations of anxiety and crisis and tension, men reacted in certain ways and some of these ways they found satisfying. Those ways of acting which they found satisfying became habitual and hardened into ritual, and dogmas and beliefs were later put forward to explain and justify the ritual practices. According to this view, the reason why certain forms of activity have 'caught on', become ritual, and got a wide currency, is that they brought brought comfort and eased tension. Because they gave comfort and eased tension, they were believed to bring about the effects which those who practised them desired, and the stronger the belief in their efficacy the more comfort they gave.

According to one form of this theory, it is the emotions to which the collective performance of the ritual gives rise which are the source of the sense of the supernatural. Those who take this view believe that there are no gods, and that God is merely the symbol for society, and religious ritual the symbolic enactment of certain relations between the individual and society. But these are deep subjects which I have no space to discuss. In any case, origins are shrouded in the mists of antiquity, and perhaps no useful purpose is served by asking which of the three elements in religion—beliefs, ritual practices and emotional attitudes—came first. What we can say is that wherever we find religion we find some measure of all three. They interact and mutually modify and support one another.

To me, the form of the theory which derives the sense of the supernatural from society and social sentiments seems to reverse the natural order of things. For men come together and co-operate in ritual activities for specific purposes and on special occasions, such as hunting game, or growing crops or protecting themselves. They do not come together merely or even mainly for performing ritual or religious practices; and social cohesion and collective sentiments of mutual goodwill seem to be the results or the fruits of ritual activities directed to other ends, rather than themselves the sources from which religious and ritual activities arise. I would, however, admit that the instrumental or practical uses of ritual are secondary to its expressive use. But I cannot pursue here these interesting but difficult questions.

In conclusion, I should like to note that while ritual has its uses, it has also its dangers. Its appeal is mainly to one side of our nature—the non-rational and especially the emotional side; and emotions are in danger of running to excess unless they are restrained and checked by rational and reflective considerations. Though we regard the situations to which ritual is the response and the ends to which it is the means as of profound import-ance, our ideas regarding them and their significance are vague and indefinite, mere hints and suggestions, if even that. While it may be impossible to get very clear ideas about them, it is desirable that we should make our ideas about them as clear as possible, and that we should subject them and their ritual expression to the scrutiny of reason. Otherwise, we are in danger of being carried away into all sorts of emotional extravagances and of mistaking myths and metaphors for literal reality.

This is especially liable to happen when the emotions are collective, as in certain forms of political ritual. It may well be true that the creative and formative aspects of our nature are in danger of being restricted or repressed by the rigidity of clear concepts, but the danger of being carried away by feelings stimulated by vague and amorphous ideas to which we attach a profound significance is no less great. The collective emotions which are aroused when men engage together in certain forms of political or religious ritual may engender moral fervour, but they do not give light or guidance. As Whitehead puts it, 'Intense emotions are evidence of some vivid experience, but they are a poor guarantee of its correct interpretation.' 'Thus', he continues, 'the dispassionate criticism of religious beliefs is beyond all things necessary.' And this is even more true of political beliefs and ritual. Life needs direction as well as drive, and neither of these will perform the functions of the other. It should, however, be added that part of the value of a well-established ritual is that it provides an opportunity for the orderly expression of strong and conflicting emotions and tends to prevent them from running riot.

I might sum up my main conclusions thus: Ritual is necessary to express experiences and attitudes which cannot be adequately expressed in any other way; to communicate emotional experiences which cannot be directly conveyed to others; to keep such experiences alive because emotions are fleeting; to awaken them when they are absent and cannot be recalled at will; to restrain them and canalize them into appropriate forms; to communicate the significance of situations which seem important, but of which the significance cannot be adequately expressed in conceptual terms; to give men spiritual support and to enable them to act appropriately in situations, such as the presence of the supernatural, which they do not understand and cannot control.

The effect of taking part together in ritual activities is to promote the mental integrity of the individual and the social harmony of the group, and to produce a spirit of mutual trust and goodwill which overflows into all the activities of life and enables people to undertake their ordinary activities and to face the hazards and hardships of life with renewed vigour and confidence. But ritual activities will produce these beneficial results only so long as those who engage in them believe in their efficacy: not their efficacy to produce these results, but their efficacy, for example, to bring strength and security and good fortune and to put people into a proper relation to the supernatural.

Constitution Making

W. J. M. MACKENZIE

Professor of Government, University of Manchester

I IMAGINE THAT my part in this symposium is to discuss the type of relationships which we commonly call political. This is an ocean of debate, and it is unwise to set out on it without plotting a course. I want therefore to choose one train of thought about political organization and to stick to it fairly closely.

Probably the common idea of politics includes two types of relationship which are both present in our minds and are difficult to bring together in a coherent scheme: on the one hand, power and the struggle for power; on the other hand, a constitution, the idea of legitimate power or power self-limited through a choice of institutions. The contrast is familiarly expressed in the phrase, 'A government of laws, and not of men', which has a pretty continuous history in the West since the contrast was drawn between Greeks and Barbarians in the fifth century before Christ.[1]

For various reasons I wish to deal mainly with the second type of relationship, that concerned with forms of government; first, because this fits in best with what Professor Macbeath has written about ritual; second, because I am rather tired of what

[1] The line is first clearly drawn by Aeschylus and Herodotus—see in particular the words which Herodotus gives to the Spartan king in exile who was with the Persians at the Hellespont and before Thermopylae (*Herodotus*, VII, 114 and 209).

passes for a tough-minded attitude in academic discussions of politics. Between the wars we were all disillusioned with the idea that we could by reason discover the best form of government: we were inclined (I speak in terms of my own experience) to think that it was more logical to begin by searching not for the springs of virtue, but for the springs of power. After all, there were so many things that could be done to make the world better—if only one had the power. This was a natural reaction from the type of constitution-making rather unfairly called Wilsonian; it could draw to its support all sorts of persuasive analogies from natural science; and it coincided with a short period (the only one) when Marxism had some real life in it as a political theory in this country.[1]

More recent experience has reinstated an older commonplace, that the real problems of reform begin only when the reformers have gained power; and there has been an equally strong reaction against very simple scientific analogies, which led us to talk of political power as if it were a substance or form of energy which could be stored in tanks or batteries and drawn upon at need by the man who knew the switch. The common idea now is that power is social and not individual; that it is intelligible only as one type of relationship within a system which exists apart from individuals and dictates rôles to all individuals, including the most powerful. Social anthropology would, I suppose, admit the existence of temporary and unstable power held by an individual, but only as a transitional phase which must end quite quickly either in destruction or a return to stability. The modern commonplace is (in other language) very similar to that to which Dicey referred when he was explaining the real limits on the theoretical power of Parliament: 'The Soldan of Egypt, or the Emperor of Rome, might drive his harmless subjects, like brute beasts, against their sentiments and inclination: But he must, at least, have led his *mamalukes*, or *praetorian bands* like men, by their opinion.'[2]

[1]One might call this period 'middle Laski': but Laski himself was never wholly absorbed in it, because he brought with him so much from nineteenth century Oxford and from pluralism.

[2]Dicey, *Law of the Constitution*, eighth ed., p. 75, quoting Hume *Essays*, I(1875 ed.), pp. 109–10.

This puts the matter in an individualist frame of reference, not a sociological one, but the implication is much the same in the language of the eighteenth century or of the twentieth. All political institutions work in much the same way, and the practical differences between them lie outside politics, in the personality of the ruler or the tone of the culture. This is the theme of the 'Trimmer' in all ages:—

> *For forms of government let fools contest:*
> *What'er is best administered is best,*

as Pope wrote,[1] echoing the language of those, such as Temple and Halifax, who helped to drive 'enthusiasm' out of fashion in the last years of the seventeenth century. This may be the right answer in the twentieth century too: I have nothing against it except that while it denies the possibility of political programmes, it is itself a programme. In fact, it sets on one side the thing that we first look for when we set out to study politics. The impulse to study politics is an impulse to improve institutions; it can make no headway unless it contrives first to understand existing institutions, but it cannot stop there. The presupposition of political study is that men are not simply moulded by institutions, but can by intelligence and effort make better institutions for themselves. This is not (I think) a presupposition that can be proved, indeed it is a fertile mother of paradoxes: but we cannot abandon it without a good deal of embarrassment here and now. After all, the British are professional constitution-makers for others if not for themselves, as one can see in news about the colonies from one day to the next. This is an important invisible item in our balance of payments, and one in which political scientists cannot help getting involved. That is one personal reason why I prefer to start from the problem of constitution-making, rather than from the problem of power.

Let me next narrow the issue still further. One meets oppressive paradoxes at once if one makes a frontal attack on the problem of making political institutions in existing States, or in the colonies, or between States; but no one doubts that administrative institutions are made every day, and that they

[1] *Essay on Man*, Epistle III, lines 303-4.

can be better or worse made. The Science of Administration is rather too pompous a name for our limited knowledge about these things, but no one doubts that an army or a Ministry must have defined ranks, and defined duties, and a regular procedure for doing business; Weber makes rather too much of it, but no one doubts that hierarchical organization is an invention, not a spontaneous growth, and that it has been as important as mechanical inventions like the lever or the wheel.

In the last fifty years administrative science has gone through the same phases as political science. It began with easy optimism about the possibility of improvement by reorganization—'rationalization' as it was called in the 1920s, a period not otherwise noted for its rationalism. There was then a reaction into extreme scepticism about the importance of hierarchical organization. The contrast between formal and informal organization was beginning to be popular before 1939, but its vogue was spread by the experience of dons and authors in the civil service and the armed forces. It was a shock to learn by experience that there were actually people living behind the great façade of bureaucratic organization in the Ministries and in the Army, and that business was done there, much as in the outer world, by winning friends and influencing people: perhaps in a more primitive way, because the bureaucratic economy runs without money, and if one wants service from a colleague one cannot get it by paying for it in cash. This is the theme of that fine book, *The Small Back Room*, and of some good stories about the forces: it has also got into the text-books, and there, I think, it has been overdone.[1] A good many students must go out with the idea that it really does not matter about organization in an office or a factory, because everything depends on human relations; in Biblical terms, 'The letter killeth, but the spirit giveth life'. St. Paul exaggerates, and so did Elton Mayo, though his language was more cautious; the letter of the law may sometimes kill, but it is rarely irrelevant.

Let us then look rather briefly at the rôle of formal organization in the place where it is strongest, the hierarchical structure

[1] This has been largely an American trend, and the Americans are now coming to the same conclusion about it: see (for instance) Arthur W. Macmahon, *Administration in Foreign Affairs* (University of Alabama, 1953), at p.168.

of bureaucracy, and let us see what sort of thing it is. And do not think I am forgetting the importance of human relations because I say little about them here.

The bureaucratic situation is dominated by a formal code called 'The Regulations'—perhaps most people know best the initials K.R. and A.C.I., but a similar code is implicit in any rational organization of this type. 'The Regulations' are the central paradox, to which we must return later; under shelter of this paradox reign order and reason. Perhaps we can analyse the system in four ways:—

1. The structure of ranks and posts: in sociological jargon, a formalized status system, defining grades, qualifications, and privileges.

2. The distribution of duties; the forms of specialization defined as it were perpendicularly and laterally, so as to settle the functions of each branch and post and to define the powers of decision at each level. This produces the familiar genealogical tree of his office organization which is engraved on the heart of every competent bureaucrat.

3. Procedures, or what the efficiency men call a 'flow-chart': the rules which state the routes by which different types of business are to 'flow' through the office, and the sort of *imprimatur* to be set on business at each stage, so that it may pass on to the next stage, and finally attain the beatitude of decision. Once upon a time the suppliant member of the public 'flowed' through the office himself, paying the proper fee to the proper official whose business it was to attach the proper seal at each point of sorting. Now, documents flow unsupported and the public pay their fees in taxation and not across the desk. But the principle is the same: the proper persons must say the proper things in the proper order, or the decision will be invalid—to speak strictly, there will be no true decision at all.

4. It may be well to add (finally) a fourth category of regulations: a very important category, but not on quite the same footing as the first three. The first three define what the office is: the fourth category tells it what it is to do. The first three are constitutional laws; the fourth is a sort of generalized command. Here one is concerned with a hierarchy of action, not

with a hierarchy of posts: a line of action is given from outside the organization in very general terms, at each official level it is narrowed down by regulation or precedent, till it reaches finally the lowest official and the lowest point, where the general becomes the particular, and the official is in theory no more than a rubber-stamp in the hand of the master of the organization. I say 'in theory', to emphasize that this is only one side of the story; an official may be given no official discretion to grant your request, but no one can take away his human discretion to be surly or courteous, or perhaps even to give a hint that if you could change one or two points of no substance to you it would be possible for him to agree after all.

Bureaucratic regulations thus imply two hierarchies, a hierarchy of men, or rather of men playing official parts, and a hierarchy of action. It is scarcely necessary to illustrate that these are interdependent; you cannot pursue a policy rationally unless you have a rational organization—and the organization is form without meaning unless it is there to execute a policy.[1] From this one can go on to work out quite plausible and useful doctrines about types of organization in relation to types of action; up to a point this can be done *a priori* as a kind of logical exercise, but to bring it down to earth one must relate theories about organization to the conditions of any given society. The matter then becomes more confusing.

For instance, good organizations work much more by teamwork than by command, and one can work out some general theories about the two things: but in practice teamwork is largely developed by training under strict command, and as teamwork develops it displaces command, even though the command structure is kept in reserve for emergencies. Again, it is obvious that an organization cannot be better than the men who make it up, and at first they are raw material given to the organizer by the general condition of society. But an organiza-

[1] A similar point is made on p. 1 of Professor Macmahon's *Administration in Foreign Affairs*; and since writing this I have noticed that Kurt Lewin applies this analogy of 'hierarchy of purpose' to distinguish the adult personality from that of the child. (*Field Theory in Social Science*, Tavistock Publications, 1952, at pp. 102 and 110).

tion in using men changes them, so that they diverge in many ways from the rest of society and become a new social type within it: the organization creates a new social world of its own.

These are puzzles which need to be handled carefully both in theory and in practice, but they do not make it impossible to argue rationally about (for instance) the best form of organization for some particular purpose in Britain at the present day: the 'science of administration' or management has often made itself absurd by claiming too much, but it would be just as absurd to claim too little. It is really obvious that in any given situation different types of formal organization will have different effects on people and on action; that some people know a good deal about this; and that with due precaution it is possible to analyse their experience in general terms. This is constitution-making as practised daily at every level of society, from the school, the football-team and the factory to Ministries and nationalized industries; and I am anxious to maintain that this sort of constitution-making is a rational operation—that by taking thought we can improve our administrative efficiency, or our dividends, or our chances of winning the World Cup.

I have called this 'constitution-making': the next thing is to consider whether the analogy is fair, and whether from relatively optimistic conclusions about the science of administration one can draw any conclusions at all about the science of politics, taking that to mean the idea of self-knowledge and self-improvement in politics.[1] The analogy can of course be followed for some distance without serious difficulty. Any constitution is in part a 'distribution of duties'; for instance, it establishes posts such as those of President or Minister or Member of Parliament and assigns duties to them, and 'organic laws' (as the French call this type of constitutional law) may regulate these things in detail. Indeed, the line between organic law and administrative law is so fine as to be imperceptible: certainly, one can criticize a constitution with reference to

---

[1] Sir Ivor Jennings, *The Law and the Constitution*, 3rd ed. (1943) at p. 314: 'The people in a democracy are free to learn what facts they please about their own system of government, and *to change it if they can think of a better*'. (my italics). This seems a perfect illustration of the theme and its paradoxes.

purpose as freely as one can administration—subject always to agreement about what the constitution is for.[1]

This proviso throws into relief the difference between politics and administration. The latter is protected from political reality by the myth of 'the Regulations': the world rests on an elephant, the elephant on a tortoise, the tortoise on what? The Regulations rest on the Minister, the Minister on Parliament, Parliament on the Constitution, the Constitution on what? It would be logical to break off here and to ask for a definition of Constitution; this is a dilemma of the Hare and Tortoise type, and as Professor Ryle has been pointing out recently, this sort of puzzle generally arises from ambiguities in definition. There is certainly ambiguity in our use of the word 'constitution'; some people take it to mean a document of a particular kind, others to mean a political system, and trouble arises if the two senses are combined.[2] But it is not easy to suggest a new formula or a compromise formula without doing violence to the goddess Constitution (constitutions have been deified before now), so that I should prefer to proceed by suggesting elements which go together in the ordinary confused idea of a constitution.

To one of these I have alluded, the element of bureaucratic organization. This is important because orderly procedure is very valuable both for efficiency and for sentiment: but it is not the heart of the matter. I think three other elements have to be added.

The first is that a constitution implies a state: do not take this in too literal a sense, but it is perhaps the most recognizable way of saying that one cannot talk about a constitution for very long without raising difficult questions about political entities.

[1]Sir Ivor Jennings, *op. cit.* at p. 131: 'As in the creation of law, the creation of a convention must be due to the reason of the thing, because it accords with the prevailing political philosophy'. Jennings, who is in principle a 'constitution-maker', though a cautious one, is here trying boldly to absorb conventions (generally supposed to be irrational) into a rational structure of politics.

[2]Professor Wheare (*Modern Constitutions*, p. 3) chooses the former; Sir Ivor Jennings is close to the latter; but neither contrives to be quite consistent or free from paradox.

The problem of sovereignty became a bore in the hands of the Benthamites and the British Hegelians, and in the 1930s one's heart warmed to Sir Ivor Jennings when he wrote the whole thing off as a 'politico-theological dogma'.[1] But the dogma comes to life again as soon as one tries to talk analytically about some very practical problems of our own day: for instance, the clauses in the South African constitution which protect the 'coloured' vote, or the French attitude to the proposal for a European Defence Community, or the limits of action against political suspects in a liberal democracy. One cannot press very hard on the dry forms of constitutional law without touching the naked nerve of personal allegiance and individual decision.

The second point is that all constitutions contain an element of description. This is most obvious when one considers a constitution like the British constitution which is in the technical sense 'unwritten'; there is no document called 'The Constitution'. The nearest to it that one can find is a book by Bagehot called *The English Constitution*, and another by Sir Ivor Jennings called *The British Constitution*—books that claim to be about what the British do in politics, and what they feel they ought to do. In this sense the British constitution is the political sociology[2] of the British; this seems plain enough in this extreme case, but would it not be absurd to say this of a document like the American constitution, or of a newly made constitution like that of Nigeria or British Central Africa? I must beware of a play on words, but I think I can make the point quite fairly in two ways.

In a sense, the American constitution is, as Bryce said,[3] a document that 'may be read through aloud in twenty-three minutes', and the document is law, not description. But what political meaning could the document have for someone who read it for the first time with no knowledge of America and no knowledge of the political tradition within which it was written? The American constitution has meaning only as a document in its setting; a political system, expounded to us by great writers, in which this document is a central point for

[1] *op. cit.* at p. 148.
[2] Or even 'political ecology'.
[3] *The American Commonwealth* (1915 ed.) vol. I, p. 374.

loyalties and struggles for power. One can put this in another way, if one looks at constitutions newly framed by the lawyers, which have had no time to acquire associations and tacit understandings, and which seem like new structures in an old landscape. Undoubtedly, the constitution-maker has a wide range of choice, but his choice is not infinite: he will not make a real constitution unless he uses a working political language and embodies in institutions the situation as it exists. A lawyer's constitution is dead until it strikes roots in the political soil; and it will not do so unless it contains an element of what I called above "political sociology". There are plenty of constitutions in the books which are no more than sham constitutions because their authors disregarded this, often deliberately and for objects of their own.

The third element is that a constitution has sanctity. In the Latin tag, *numen inest*; the language is vague, but its vagueness is less confusing than the apparent precision of language about norms and value-judgements, and about the difference between statements of fact and statements of value. One of the puzzles about constitutions is that a statement of fact is also a statement of value: a record of how men have behaved is a statement about how they ought to behave. Men seem to switch easily from one mood to the other, and even to use both together: a constitution has got to be on both sides of the fence at once, to be both political sociology and political ethics.

This way to put it may be confusing; but it seems less confusing than to put the point by emphasizing that a constitution is law. I think this is true, and that all law ultimately faces the dilemma posed by the idea of constitutional law.[1] If a constitution is law, then it is law made by an authority which the law creates; the circle cannot be broken except by postulating a *Grundnorm* as the formal origin of the lawyer's system—a solution consistent in itself which frees the lawyer by transferring the problem to other disciplines which are no better equipped to handle it.

However, the paradox is acceptable enough to common sense. A people creates itself by its capacity to recognize com-

[1]Appendix III to Jennings, *The Law and the Constitution*, is much concerned with this point. Cf. A. F. Bentley, *The Process of Government* at p. 295.

mon imperatives and to respect them. This is very loose language, but it seems to have a recognizable political meaning. For instance, there was a period after the French Revolution when the old regimes tried to compromise with the new by offering what was called a Charter or constitution '*octroyée*'—something given by the King's grace to his people. In France, the legitimist constitution of 1814 was not very different from the Orleanist constitution of 1830, except that it was enacted as of right by the people of France, not granted by the grace by 'me, Louis XVIII' to 'our people'—the 'Roi des Français' was substituted for the 'Roi de France'. The point may seem trivial: but if one is to fight for principles, this is as good a one as any on which to take a stand. The tradition of the constitution is that by it free men limit themselves, under God and the law, but under no man.[1]

One effect of proceeding in this way is to sophisticate somewhat the traditional Western distinction between true and false forms of government, and perhaps to endanger it. The distinction between democracy and dictatorship has become a nuisance, because it is so easy to twist to fit any case; but at best it was a feeble substitute for the older distinction between governments under law and governments that know no law— between constitutional government and oriental despotism.[2] This is a fortress worth defending; it may seem to weaken it if one proceeds by taking constitution and State to be corelatives, and insisting that a true constitution is both descriptive and imperative. This may have awkward consequences. For instance, has the U.S.S.R. a constitution in this sense? To begin with, there is a written and enacted document, the Stalin Constitution of 1936, as later amended. One should not assume offhand that this is wholly a sham, for it was composed by clever men, and there were certainly some things in it intended to command wide allegiance in Russia. Nevertheless the document is largely futile both as a description of Russian government and as a set of rules respected by Russian leaders.

[1] The point is neatly made by the amendment which in 1925 added a new first section to the South African constitution, 'The people of the Union acknowledge the sovereignty and guidance of Almighty God.'

[2] As characterized by Montesquieu: e.g., *Esprit des Lois*, bk. 3, chap. V.

Is there then a real Russian constitution behind the sham? Is there a constitution which binds the Mamalukes who are led "like men by their opinions"? I do not know: but I think that this is in principle an answerable question. It may be that at the centre is an anarchy like that of Hitler's court. Or it may be that there are a set of rules well understood by those who hold power: that the struggles of the ambitious are conducted within limits set by the beliefs of followers, on whom they are dependent. If the latter is true, I should feel inclined to say that there is a true Russian (or "Communist," or what you will) state; that it has a true constitution; and that it is in consequence formidable, because it is, in its own sense, government under law.

Hitler's Germany broke down largely because Hitler ranted about the unity of Germans, but had no conception of unity in government; indeed, his art of despotism was to break unity wherever he saw it, and in breaking unity he isolated himself from the advice of almost all able men. It may be that in the end the U.S.S.R. will break in the same way, but we should be fools to assume lightly that this is not a stable regime and a true state, although an oligarchic one. Nor should it be assumed on the other side, because France, or the U.S.A., has the traditions of a state and is arrayed in all the verbiage of constitutionalism, that a true state and a true constitution exist. Lincoln remarked in his First Inaugural Address,[1] at the outset of the Civil War:—

> 'A majority held in restraint by constitutional checks and limitations, and always changing easily with deliberate changes of popular opinions and sentiments, is the only true sovereign of a free people. Whoever rejects it does, of necessity, fly to anarchy or to despotism'.

'Anarchy' is as destructive of constitutional government as is 'despotism'.

I have referred to four aspects of a constitution: it is an administrative structure, it is a description of a political situation, it has binding force, and it is a *supreme* set of rules, the articulation of a political entity—'the supreme law of the land'. Let me now work back to the problem of constitution-making;

[1]Everyman Library edition of the *Speeches and Letters* at p. 171.

this goes on all the time in the British Commonwealth, and the possibility of it is one of the assumptions of our scheme of things. So one has strong inducements to be optimistic.

First, the political situation and its relation to the social structure. This seems to be outside our power; indeed, one certain recipe for failure is to assume facts out of existence. It is true that aspirations and loyalties are facts: it is true, as John Stuart Mill says, that 'one person with a belief is a social power equal to ninety-nine who have only interests'.[1] But this is not to the point unless the one man in a hundred exists and can be found.

Second, the mechanical construction of political institutions is no harder than the mechanical construction of administrative institutions, provided that we know and face the facts, and provided that we know what we are trying to do. This last is a large limitation because it throws us back upon the hardest question, that of political entity. How can a people have a purpose? And if they have one, how can they know authoritatively what it is except through institutions set up in the light of their purpose—to tell them what their purpose is? I do not think the logicians have yet got to work on the logic of the first person plural, but a layman may guess that it is not the same as that of the first person singular.

The dilemmas set by the idea of men acting freely yet in unity are well known: and no one is likely to produce an easy answer to them. However, they are no worse for men acting together in politics than for men acting together in any other capacity: common purpose and joint action are ideas that we have to live with, and it is not really in doubt that individuals can help or hinder the growth of this free unity, and can do it consciously. I do not say that any single man can *make* it— to do so would be to pile contradiction on contradiction, because the unity in question is jointly made and self-made. But it is a recognizable fact of politics, or of day-to-day life, that some individuals can help more than others, because they are wiser or because they try harder. Here I agree entirely with what M. Bertrand de Jouvenel said in a distinguished lecture last year:[2] this is a supreme art. But I do not like his

[1] *Considerations on Representative Government* (1861 ed.), p. 14.
[2] Published as 'The Nature of Politics', *Cambridge Journal*, May 1954.

conclusion that this art is the supreme object of political science, as Machiavelli perhaps also thought in his passion for the unity of Italy.

For one thing, this flatters the vanity of politicians too much: there may be one man here and there who touches the hidden springs of politics and gets the result that he expects—but most politicians are representatives, not leaders; it is easier to be a good representative than a good leader, and a great deal more useful than to be a bad leader. Besides, the academic student cannot say much more about the supreme art of politics than about the supreme arts of music or poetry. One can define the limiting factors, one can trace the history of the idiom common to all performers, great and small, but one cannot capture the essence of the great man's art. If this can be done at all it is a job for artists, not for scholars: Thucydides on Pericles, Vergil on Augustus, even Walt Whitman on Lincoln. But the charm of artists may be as dangerous as the vanity of politicians, and I am not very anxious to cement the alliance.

Nevertheless, I think one must stand firm at this central point: the making of unity is not wholly a social process or even one of joint will—individual will and wisdom are vital to it. If we pass this point, we are on easier ground. The third element to which I referred was that of the sanctity of the constitution, and here I must in large part refer you to what has been written by Professor Macbeath. A constitution purports to be a rational structure: indeed the whole notion of government under law belongs to the same realm of ideas as right reason, natural law, and the equality of men in so far as they realize their nature as men. Constitutions purport to be as rational as bureaucracies, but like them they live by myth-making and ritual. Rational organization breeds repetition, repetition breeds habit, and habit breeds affection. An action originally purposive is in the end performed for its own sake: and in the process there grow up on the one hand 'rationalizations', in the new sense of false explanations, on the other hand unexpected effects which may often be good effects.

In a bureaucracy a piece of procedure may be well designed for a particular purpose at a particular time: times change, the procedure goes on: someone asks questions, and angry defenders think of justifications for the *status quo*. These are often so silly that they hasten reform: and reform may take place without much thought about the problem of whether the old operation, in losing a purpose, had gained a function. Survivals may have functions even in a bureaucracy: no one really doubts that they have functions in a constitution. The Coronation itself contained, from the first, elements purely religious, and is therefore not a good case to take: but the meeting of an enlarged Privy Council which greets the Sovereign on his or her accession has no religious implications, and yet seems a fair case of constitutional ritual. This can happen equally well with a more formal constitution such as that of the United States; the rubbish, if I may so term it, about the elected electors who elect the President serves no useful purpose, but we could not abolish these gentlemen without a good deal of disturbance to the American way of life.

I am not sure that a constitution can exist at all on a scale as large as that of a nation without this element of civil ritual, which seems mere gibberish except in so far as we find false rationalizations for it. It is hard to imagine a constitution without ritual: and yet ritual cannot be enacted. Or can it? It may be that one can enact, not ritual, but ways of acting likely to give rise to ritual, as we try to do when we impose the odd routines of Westminster on the Parliaments of West Africa. Certainly there is no other way to enact sanctity: legal safeguards written into the text of a constitution have no power other than the power of myth.

The Background of Buddhism

A. L. BASHAM

Reader in Ancient Indian History, School of Oriental and African Studies, London

I WANT TO BEGIN by explaining certain ideas which you will find implicitly or explicitly expressed in much Indian thought on religion and metaphysics, especially the idea of two levels of truth. On the ordinary everyday plane, there is pragmatic truth, which is simple and obvious. I am here now, a real person writing in a real room. But there is also an ultimate truth, and what is thought to be the ultimate truth may vary considerably from sect to sect. For instance, the most important school of Hindu metaphysics, the school known as Vedanta, teaches that I and my room and the town where I live are all part of a great cosmic illusion, and that only one impersonal spirit fills the eternity of space and time.

So we must bear in mind that, from the Indian point of view, there are two levels of truth. A further point which is not often recognized is that in Indian thought what Western logicians call the law of the excluded middle, either 'a' or not 'a', is not so rigidly applied as in Europe. On one level this exists and on one it does not. It is and it is not simultaneously. We must keep this point in mind, too, when we discuss some of the strange paradoxes of early Buddhism, especially in connexion with the concept of Nirvāna and the chain of transmigration. These paradoxes may not have appeared so paradoxical in the days and in the land in which they were first uttered.

Of course, this Indian concept of levels of truth is by no

75

means unknown in the West. It is quite a commonplace nowadays that on the practical, pragmatic level my pen is solid and more or less homogeneous matter, but according to the truth of the physicist it is just a complex pattern of particles or centres of force very sparsely scattered, with great areas of empty space between them. It is not for me to say which truth is the truer, but of course the Indian thinker had no doubts that his religious truth was fundamentally more true than the practical everyday truth.

Now a few words on the historical background of Buddhism. I am primarily a historian, and not a philosopher or expert on religion as such, and so I must fit my subject into its social and historical context.

The religion of Buddhism emerged at a time when civilization was advancing in India, and when the area of civilized culture was rapidly expanding. From the tenth to the seventh centuries B.C. the main focus of religious thought and activity had been the great sacrificial rituals, very expensive and complicated. It was believed that the world was created as the result of a great primal sacrifice at the beginning of time, when the high god, Prajāpati, offered himself to himself, priest, victim and divinity being mystically identified; and it was further believed that by the repetition of sacrifice and the immolation of numerous animals, the cosmic process was maintained, and that without sacrifice chaos would come again in the universe, and the gods themselves would perish. The sacrifice could be performed only by highly trained priests who knew the ritual in complete exactitude, the Brahmans. The Brahmans, of course, were more powerful than the gods themselves, because by their ministrations the gods were supported and maintained.

From perhaps about 700 B.C. there was a reaction against this sacrificial mysticism, and at about the same time a new idea seems to have swept like wildfire over the upper crust of Indian society, the intellectuals of the time. It may have risen from the bottom, among the lower orders, but to discuss its origin is not my purpose.

Earlier it had been believed that, when a man died, he either went to a heaven comparable to the Nordic Valhalla, where he feasted and enjoyed himself indefinitely, or, if he had not lived according to the ways of the Aryan, he went down to a miserable underground sheol, where he eked out a tenuous and gloomy half-existence, again indefinitely. But very quickly the idea of transmigration spread. There was death even in heaven; a man would be reborn again and again and his future lot would be conditioned by his present behaviour. Human beings, gods, demons, animals, even plants, were all brought into the scheme. They all had souls which transmigrated in obedience to regular laws, and their migrations were conditioned, according to most sects, by their behaviour.

This doctrine of transmigration, *Samsāra* in Sanskrit, has been a feature of nearly all Indian religious thought from that day to this, and certainly it must have met the psychic needs of important sections of the population or it would not have taken root so quickly; but to many of the best minds of the times it was acutely grievous and distasteful. They believed in it implicitly and the thought of it was very terrible to them. Since then, one of the chief religious quests of India has been to find a means of escape from transmigration, this dreary, mono-tonous round of birth and death and rebirth, which goes on and on and on. This quest, in its earliest manifestation, produced the wonderful mystical texts known as the Upanishads, which were incorporated into the canon of orthodox Vedic literature, but it also produced many heterodox sects, chief of which was that of Buddhism, which was founded in the sixth century B.C. by Siddhārtha Gautama, generally referred to by his title 'Buddha' or 'the Buddha', the 'awakened', 'he who has awakened from sleep'.

I must disclaim any attempt to discuss what the Buddha really taught. Among Buddhologists, if I can coin a word, there is no consensus whatever on this question. The general view is that we do not know and we probably never shall know what the Buddha really taught, though some authorities have put forward pet theories. All we can say is that there was a historical Buddha, but that the sayings attributed to him are, in many cases, much later. In fact, the teaching of the historical Buddha is far more uncertain than is the teaching of the historical Jesus according to left-wing protestant theologians.

And so we must be quite clear that what I speak of is not the teachings of Buddha but the teachings of Buddhism, and when I say 'Buddha said', that is really a figure of speech. I mean 'early Buddhism taught'.

It is well known that there are two chief branches of Buddhism, with doctrines differing in many particulars; they are the Lesser and the Greater Vehicles, *Hīnayāna* and *Mahāyāna*. The terminology was devised by the Greater Vehicle and it implies that the Lesser Vehicle is capable of carrying only a few beings to Salvation, whereas the Greater Vehicle can carry a large number. It is a thorny question among the authorities as to which of the two branches preserves the more reliable historical tradition, but certainly as far as dogma and doctrine is concerned the Lesser Vehicle is more authentic. Its scriptures are positively older than those of the Greater Vehicle. The two are perhaps very roughly comparable to Protestantism and Roman Catholicism, with the difference that the less ritualistic sect in Buddhism is the older. In the Lesser Vehicle there is only one surviving school, the Theravāda, which is prevalent in Ceylon, Burma, Thailand, Cambodia and Laos. In the Greater Vehicle there are numerous sects now prevalent in China, Japan and Tibet, some of which originated in India and some as local developments. The schism arose after very early divergencies and became virtually final in the first centuries of the Christian era. There are many differences, the main one being the concept of the Bodhisattva, which I shall touch on later.

According to the tradition, the Buddha set himself a definite problem, and the whole religion is based on his solution of that problem. In this Buddhism differs from most other religions, which define Man's relations with the power or powers which govern the universe, and instruct him on how he should conduct himself in relation to those powers. Buddhism is much more limited in essence. Questions such as whether the world is eternal or not and how it came into being were, according to the Buddha, of no great importance. They were useless; it was not worth while wasting time upon them. The really important question is not cosmological or metaphysical, but rather psychological: Why does man suffer? Why is he unhappy? 'As the ocean has only one flavour, the flavour of salt,' said the Buddha, 'so has my teaching only one flavour, the flavour of sorrow and the cessation of sorrow'. The word which I translate 'sorrow' is the Sanskrit *duḥkha*, which has a much wider connotation. All unpleasant states of mind and sensations, dissatisfaction, boredom, depression, misery, are included in this one term.

When a man is wounded by an arrow, we are told, one does not worry about such questions as who made the arrow, or what flights it has, or what metal goes to make its tip, or even why it was shot; the important thing is to remove the arrow and bandage the wound. In later Buddhism, especially in the Greater Vehicle, there was much metaphysical thought and speculation but metaphysics is not the kernel of Buddhist, teaching.

According to the tradition, the Buddha was the son of a great king; in fact, he was the son of a small tribal chieftain; he left his father's palace and wandered for six years from hermit to hermit, seeking an answer to his question, 'Why does man suffer?' One day, when he was almost in despair at not finding the answer, he sat down under a great *pīpal* tree, near the city of Gayā, and resolved that he would not get up until he found the truth. After sitting for forty-nine days in meditation, he found a solution to his own satisfaction. Then he got up and walked to the city of Banaras, some 150 miles away, and there he found in a grove outside the city five former ascetic colleagues of his, to whom he preached his first sermon, which is the basic doctrine of all Buddhist sects. I will read you a somewhat abridged version of this—the *Dhamma-cakka-pavattana-sutta*, or Sermon of the Turning (or Setting in Motion) of the Wheel of the Law. The translation is my own:—

'Thus I have heard; once the Master was at Banaras at the deer park called Isipatana. There the Master addressed the Five Monks as follows: There are two ends not to be served by a wanderer. What are those two? The pursuit of desires and the pleasure which springs from desires, which is base, common, leading to rebirth, ignoble and unprofitable; and the pursuit of pain and hardship, which is grievous, ignoble and unprofitable. The Middle Way of the Tathāgata (one of the

Buddha's titles) avoids both these ends. It is enlightened, it brings clear vision, it makes for wisdom and it leads to peace, insight, full wisdom, and Nirvāna. What is this Middle Way? It is the Noble Eightfold Path—right views, right resolve, right speech, right conduct, right livelihood, right effort, right recollection and right meditation. This is the Middle Way. And this is the Noble Truth of sorrow. Birth is sorrow, age is sorrow, disease is sorrow, death is sorrow, contact with the unpleasant is sorrow, separation from the pleasant is sorrow, every wish unfulfilled is sorrow; in short, all the five components of individuality are sorrow. And this is the Noble Truth of the arising of sorrow. It arises from thirst, the craving which leads to rebirth, which brings delight and passion, and seeks pleasure, now here, now there, the thirst for sensual pleasure, the thirst for continued life, the thirst for power. And this is the Noble Truth of the stopping of sorrow. It is the complete stopping of that thirst so that no passion remains; the leaving of it, being emancipated and being released from it, giving no place to it. And this is the Noble Truth of the way which leads to the stopping of sorrow. It is that same Noble Eightfold Path, right views, right resolve, right speech, right conduct, right livelihood, right effort, right recollection and right meditation.'

The Four Noble Truths are very different indeed from comparable basic texts of other religions, such as the Ten Commandments, or the Sermon on the Mount. Nothing at all is said about the soul, nothing about God, and there is only a passing reference to the future life and the doctrine of transmigration, which was by now the fundamental presupposition of everybody. Instead, we have a series of four propositions which can be roughly paraphrased thus:—

Suffering is inevitable in ordinary human existence; it is caused by individual cravings and desires; it can be eradicted only by eradicating such desires, and this can be done only by disciplined and virtuous living and mental and psychic training.

Another old and much repeated doctrine of Buddhism, which the Buddha is also said to have realized during his meditations under the Bodhi Tree, is what is known as *Paticcasamuppāda*, the chain of dependent origination. This takes us deeper into the question of human personality and gives another complementary explanation of the mystery of suffering, but the twelve terms of the chain of the dependent origination are among the most obscure elements in Buddhist philosophy. It is doubtful whether anybody, either in the East or in the West, really understands what the Buddha, or whoever composed this chain of twelve terms, fully implied; but they appear again and again in Buddhist literature, and have been commented upon again and again and interpreted differently by many authorities, ancient and modern. I cannot claim to give a definite interpretation.

Out of ignorance arise conformations of character, thence consciousness, thence physical existence, thence the six fields of the sense organs (thought is the sixth sense in the Indian classification), thence contact, thence sensation, thence desire, thence attachment, thence becoming, thence birth, and thence come age and death, and all the ills the flesh is heir to.

These twelve are almost inexplicable, but evidently the chain implies that behind the craving and desire which cause our human misery, is another factor, a basic ignorance. The Sanskrit term is exactly cognate with the English 'unwisdom'—*avidyā*, a deep, almost instinctive, false belief in the nature of the universe.

Again, I give you another Buddhist classification. The world we know has three salient characteristics: it is sorrowful, it is transient, and it is soulless. The world is full of sorrow. As I said, the word *duhkha* has a much wider range of connotation than the English word 'sorrow'. For the ordinary mortal, sorrow cannot be escaped. We are born in sorrow, we die in sorrow, sorrow awaits us throughout our life and dogs our tracks everywhere. The main cause of our sorrow is brought out in the second characteristic of the world. The world is transient, nothing whatever lasts, you never cross the same river twice. The universe is conceived as a continuous flux of events, one causing the next in a series of innumerable, interacting chains. Yet we cannot but act on the delusion of permanence. We encounter things and we cling to them and we want to keep them, but of course by the very nature of them and ourselves, we cannot do so, and so we are haunted continuously at the bottom of our minds by the fear of having to part from them, and sooner or later they are forced from us and we suffer. We can never find eternity for our joys, and so we are in one way or another unhappy.

That is a very grim doctrine when looked at from the negative aspect in which Buddhism sees it, but it was put by a great English poet in a positive way which gives it a rather different complexion. I quote one of the most pregnant of William Blake's gnomic verses:—

> 'He who binds to himself a joy
> Does the winged life destroy;
> But he who kisses the joy as it flies
> Lives in eternity's sunrise.'

Thirdly, there is no soul. If the world is transient, the invididual is no different. There is no permanent, unchanging core of the personality which lasts for ever or indefinitely. The individual, like everything else in the universe, is a compound which is continually changing, and which must, sooner or later, completely alter. Here I want to return to the Sermon of the Turning of the Wheel of the Law. You will remember the phrase, 'in short all the five components of individuality are sorrow'. The five components of individuality, according to traditional Buddhist psychology, are the body, sensations, perceptions, states of mind and consciousness. These five in varying combinations make up the man. He is, in fact, an aggregate of these elements, continually altering in composition. We are told that just as the word 'chariot' is a convenient term to describe a number of pieces of wood and metal put together in a certain manner, so terms such as person, personality, soul, individual, and so on, are convenient labels for complex series of events caused by the interaction of numerous factors. The full-grown man is obviously not quite the same as the schoolboy, and the schoolboy is not quite the same person as the infant in arms. There is no reason, says Buddhism, to believe that any permanent entity is carried over from the baby to the adult. The one is caused by the other, and by the influence of various external factors. Every moment, in fact, the old man dies and the new man comes to be, caused by the one who has passed. There is no being, but only becoming.

In this connexion there is one common error about Buddhism which I should like to demolish, before I go further. Buddhism is not an atheistic religion. The Buddhism of the Greater Vehicle built up a whole new mythology of divine beings, but even the Lesser Vehicle is not atheistic. All forms of Buddhism admit the existence of mighty supernatural powers. The early Buddhist scriptures speak much of the high god, Brahmā, who presides over the universe and falsely believes that he created it, when actually it came to be through the processes of natural law. The world is full of divinities of all kinds, gods, demi-gods, and good and evil spirits; but they are all fundamentally of the same character as men, animals and plants, all liable to sorrow or dissatisfaction in some measure, all transient, though their lives are much longer than those of men; and none of them has a permanent soul. The gods themselves are merely complex chains of compounded events in the cosmic flux. They are mightier and, in general, more virtuous than we. By praying to a god we may be helped in our difficulties or we may achieve success in our ventures; but to win full and ultimate salvation the gods can help us very little. We have to stand on our own feet, and the only real help we can get from the Buddhist point of view is the inspiration of the Buddha, the Doctrine and the Order of monks, in which the believer expresses his faith in the Buddhist creed. Only they are of real use in the quest for inner peace. The only unchanging category which Buddhism of the Lesser Vehicle admits is Nirvāna. It implies a state, neither being nor not being, quite outside the universe, the blowing out of the causal process, likened to the blowing out of a lamp, the final, indescribable and inexplicable peace which comes when the individual is disintegrated.

This, then, is man according to Buddhism. What of his relationships? Man can obtain freedom from sorrow only by giving up the conviction that he is a separate, permanent entity cut off from all other entities. He must, in fact, get outside himself. He must view himself as objectively as possible from the Buddhist point of view, as a constantly changing compound, one strand in a continuously altering flux of events.

Obviously every action which is done to emphasize the individuality, to emphasize man's being completely separate from everything else, something permanent and unchanging, is bad from the Buddhist point of view. Acts of harshness, cruelty, and selfishness are, therefore, to be interpreted as frantic efforts on the part of the being who commits them to establish his illusory individuality, prompted by the often unconscious fear of union with the unpleasant or separation from the pleasant, the dread of losing what he has, or the horror of having to put up with unhappy conditions—a very deep-seated feeling, which is comparable to what German Existentialists call '*Angst*'. The bad man is so because he must futilely attempt to bind to himself the joy, instead of being content with kissing it as it flies. So the best way to happiness is altruism. There are four cardinal virtues in Buddhism, benevolence or friendship (*maitrī*, often translated love, but somewhat less emotional and less intense than the comparable Christian word in St. Paul), compassion, joy and equanimity. Notice the joy. Buddhism encourages people to be happy.

Every day the Buddhist monk is taught to meditate on these virtues and to try to develop them in himself. He must, viewing himself as from the outside, as dispassionately and objectively as possible, first feel benevolence for the bundle of ever-changing flesh and thoughts and emotions, which, on the pragmatic level of truth, he calls himself, because one cannot love others unless in the highest sense one loves oneself; and then he must mentally penetrate the whole world in all directions with the same emotion. It is believed as an article of faith by orthodox Buddhists that the daily meditations of love and compassion, joy and equanimity, of the hundreds of thousands of Buddhist monks throughout Asia, really do have a positive effect upon the welfare of the world, because these monks are every day sending out their thought-waves of goodwill—though, of course, that is purely an article of faith and we have no proof or disproof of it.

Ethically therefore, Buddhism, with its stern message of renunciation and its denial of the ultimate reality and importance of the individual, propagates much the same code—selflessness, gentleness, and kindliness in human relationships—

as do other higher religions, with their doctrines of immortal and eternal souls.

I must say a little on the developments added by the Greater Vehicle to this austere doctrine. From the point of view of the Greater Vehicle the ethics of kindliness of the Lesser Vehicle are only a higher form of selfishness, because they are directed to the selfish end of escaping the delusion of self hood. It is on this point that the schism between the Lesser and Greater Vehicles is based. According to the Lesser Vehicle, a man should attempt to gain enlightenment as quickly as possible, and the benevolence which he shows to others is something of a by-product of his efforts at working out his own salvation. The merits he gains cannot be transferred. By charity, goodness, restraint and self-control, said the Buddha, a man can store up a well-hidden treasure, a treasure which cannot be given to others and which robbers cannot steal. The only real help, other than help on the material plane, which one man can give to another, is advice and example. That is all the help the Buddha himself gave, or claimed to give. The Lesser Vehicle teaches that men should strive to become *Arhants*, 'worthies' who attain the ineffable state of Nirvāna, when their personalities virtually disintegrate. But if charity and compassion are acquired in unlimited measure in the course of this spiritual or mental development, the being who has reached a highly developed state will surely not want to pass out of the universe. Rather he will continually work for the welfare of all beings, and he will desire to be the last, rather than the first, to enter the state of final bliss.

So the sects of the Greater Vehicle introduced a new concept, the concept of the heavenly *Bodhisattva*, the being of wisdom; the term Bodhisattva occurs in the Lesser Vehicle too, but it has a different connotation which I have no time to define. With this concept there developed a whole new mythology of mighty supernatural beings, working continuously for the good of all creation, and the ideal shifted. Man must not strive so much for his own salvation as for the salvation of all things living. In the Greater Vehicle appears the idea of the transference of merit, which is foreign to the Lesser Vehicle. The truly unselfish soul voluntarily transfers the benefits and advantages, spiritual and otherwise, accruing to him from his good conduct, to the welfare of other struggling beings. Moreover, he voluntarily undertakes suffering, in the spirit of compassion for the welfare of all things living.

The text which I am going to quote now is probably from the fifth century A.D., and of course, is of the Greater Vehicle. It is part of the vow, the resolve of the Bodhisattva:—

'I take upon myself the deeds of all beings, even of those among the hells, in other worlds, in the realms of punishment. I take their suffering upon me, I bear it, I do not draw back from it, I do not tremble at it. I have no fear of it, and I do not lose heart. I must bear the burden of all beings, since I have vowed to save all things living, to bring them safe through the forest of birth, age, death and rebirth. I think not of my own salvation, but I strive to bestow on all beings the royalty of supreme wisdom. So I take upon myself the sorrows of all beings. I resolve to bear every torment in every purgatory of the universe, for it is better that I alone suffer than the multitude of living beings. I give myself in exchange. I redeem the universe from the forest of purgatory, from the womb of the flesh, from the realm of death. I agree to suffer as a ransom for all beings for the sake of all beings. Truly I will not abandon them, for I have resolved to gain supreme wisdom for the sake of all that lives, to save the world.'

Here we are very close to Christian teaching with the ideas of the Suffering Saviour, of Atonement, and of vicarious suffering, and it may well be that this doctrine entered Buddhism through the influence of Nestorianism from Persia.

Thus the Greater Vehicle reversed the direction of older Buddhism in this and in other particulars. The heavens were peopled with beneficient Bodhisattvas and Buddhas, continually working for the welfare of all things living, and the state of Nirvāna, never thoroughly defined in the Lesser Vehicle, was identified with the ultimate body of the Buddha, the supreme divine Buddha, of which the earthly historical Buddha was merely a docetic manifestation. The ultimate reality is also called the Void, Suchness, and by many other terms. In fact, it is identical with the Word Soul of most other Indian religions. And in the Greater Vehicle all beings participate in the

The Background of Buddhism

divine body of essence, the Primeval Buddha in Nirvāna, which is here and now for everybody if only they would realize it. 'The life of the world is merely a mode of Nirvāna, and there is in fact no difference between them at all', said Nārgārjuna, the greatest of the Mahāyāna philosophers. Sooner or later, all things return to the ineffable bliss of the universal essence. In one text the Buddha is said to have said that there is not one stone upon the road which will not, sooner or later, become Buddha. This mystical monism of the Greater Vehicle is completely foreign to the Lesser, but can be explained as a logical development from it.

The ethics of the abandonment of desire are, of course, primarily intended for the Buddhist Order, the monks, who give up their family ties and live together in monasteries, simply but not very austerely, to work out their salvation. This is another great misconception which prevails in the west about Buddhism. Buddhism never suggested that these austere and very difficult practices of mental training could be followed fully by the ordinary man and woman, who, for all the preaching of the Order, persistently and stubbornly refuse to give up desiring things. For the man in the street, however, there is a great deal of ethical literature, encouraging friendliness between man and man and self-sacrifice for others. Much of this is in the form of stories. We have an enormous collection of some 550 tales, the *Jātakas*, mostly based on folk stories, some very amusing, and all adapted to Buddhist purposes by making the protagonist in the story the Buddha in a former birth. In general, these stories inculcate a very high ethical standard. A man must be willing to serve other men in every way possible and to lay down his life in their service, if need be. There are also one or two important passages in the Buddhist scriptures, ascribed to the Buddha himself, which treat of human relations on the everyday level. The most striking of these is *Sigālovāda Sutta*, the sermon of admonition to Sigāla. I will conclude by quoting part of this sermon.

Sigāla is a young man who, in accordance with one of the popular religious cults of the time, is a worshipper of the six quarters. I must explain that in the traditional Indian classification the six quarters are north, south, east, west, up and down—

87

the six sides of a cube. One day the Buddha passed by when Sigāla was busily engaged in the worship of the six quarters, and politely but firmly told him that he was wasting his time. It would be far better if, instead of worshipping the six quarters, Sigāla cultivated good personal relationships in six directions; and the Buddha unfolded a remarkable series of mutual rights and duties unparalleled in any religious text I know. The most interesting of these for the twentieth century Westerner are the Buddha's instructions on the relations of husband and wife, and master and servant, which seem to foreshadow very modern ideas. Notice the wife's right to full control of domestic affairs, and to the ancient Indian counterpart of an adequate dress allowance. Notice, too, the remarkably enlightened conception of the duties of masters towards their servants, including medical attention, bonuses and regular holidays. The following translation is based on that of Dr. F. L. Woodward.

'These', said the Buddha, 'should be regarded as the six regions: mother and father are the east, teachers are the south, child and wife are the west, friends and comrades are the north, servants and workers are the below, and recluses and Brahmans are the above. Now in five ways should a son regard his parents as the east. He should say: "Supported by them as I was, I shall support them in my turn. I will do my duty by them. I will keep up the honour of my family. I will manage my inheritance and I will keep up the offerings due to relatives deceased". [This is a reference to the traditional ancestor worship in India]. And in these five ways shall mother and father, thus set in the east and ministered to by their son, show their affection from him: they should preserve him from evil; they should put him in the right way; they should have him taught a science or craft; they should provide him with a proper wife; and, in time, they should hand over their fortune to him. Thus is the eastern region protected for him, safe and free from fear.

'And in five ways, young master, should teachers be set in the south and ministered to by their pupils: by rising up to greet them, by supporting them, by readiness to learn, by ministering to them, by attentively grasping what they teach. And thus do teachers, in five ways set in the south and ministered to by their pupils, in five ways show their affection for them: they train them so that they become well-trained, they make them keep what they have learned, they are their good counsellors in every science and art, they praise them to their friends and comrades and they set up a guard for them on every side. And thus is this southern quarter protected for the Aryan and made safe and free from fear.

'And in five ways, young master, shall the wife be set in the west and ministered to by her husband: by showing her respect, by showing her compliance, by not committing adultery, by leaving her in charge, and by supplying her with finery. And in these five ways thus honoured, does she show her affection for him: by doing her duties thoroughly, by good treatment of her household, by not committing adultery, by guarding what he earns, and by skill and zeal in all she has to do. Thus is the western region protected for him, and made safe and free from fear.

'And in five ways, young master, shall friends and comrades be set in the north and ministered to by the gentleman: by charity, by kind words, by acting for their welfare, by treating them on equal terms, and by keeping one's promises to them. And in five ways do friends and comrades show their affection for the gentleman: they watch over him when he is off his guard; they watch over his property when he is off his guard; They are his refuge in time of fear; They do not forsake him in time of trouble; They show respect for the rest of his family. Thus in five ways is the northern region protected for him, and made safe and free from fear.

'And in five ways, young master, are servants and workers set in the below and ministered to by a true gentleman: he assigns them work according to their strength, he provides them with adequate food and wages, he nurses them in time of sickness, he gives them a share in any extra dainty, and in due season he gives them leave of absence. Thus do servants and workers show their affection for the true gentleman, their master: they rise up early, they take rest late, they accept what is given, they do their work thoroughly, and they praise him everywhere. And thus is the below protected, and made safe and free from fear.

'And in five ways, young master, should a gentleman seek

recluses and Brahmans [that is to say, holy men and religious teachers of all religions] in the above and minister to them: by kindly action, by kindly words, by kindly thought towards them, by not closing his doors against them, by providing for their worldly needs. And in these five ways do recluses and Brahmans show their affection for the gentleman: they restrain him from evil; they set him in the right way; they teach him what he did not know before; they clarify what he has already heard; and they show him the way to heaven. Thus in these five ways is the region above protected for him, and made safe and free from fear'.

'Thus spake the Exalted One.'

That, I think, is a very good summary of what Buddhism has to say about human relationships on the practical everyday level.

The Gospel of Truth

GILLES QUISPEL

Professor of Theology, University of Utrecht

IN 1945 SOME PEASANTS, when working on a cemetery in the neighbourhood of Nag Hammadi in Upper Egypt, discovered a jar containing thirteen codices, one of which was the Codex Jung. Most of these manuscripts belong to the Sethians, representatives of a vulgar sort of Gnosis, which seems to be older and more mythological than the Valentinian documents of the second century. Thus the background of the Gnosis of the second century becomes much clearer. Valentinus, Basilides and other learned Gnostics were rooted—it seems now—in the mythological and vulgar Gnosticism of Egypt, whose most important document, the Apocryphon of John, was also found at Nag Hammadi.

The question, where these ideas come from, cannot be answered in a satisfactory way because the new documents have not yet been published. But our evidence points in the direction of the astrology and magic of the Near East, and also of Jewish heterodoxy. Therefore the Dead Sea scrolls, the great discovery of our age, are of paramount importance also for the study of Gnosticism. The documents found in the neighbourhood of Qumran reveal to us the existence of a pre-Christian and pre-Gnostic Jewish sect. It seems by no means excluded that the origin of Gnosis is to be sought not in Greece or Iran, but in Jewish heterodoxy. An awakening sense of mythology, which was a reaction to the austere and legalistic

91

Jewish conception of monotheism, produced the first elements, or archetypal patterns, from which Gnosticism, blended with magical and astrological notions, took its course. So there is some hope that within a short time it may be possible to discern the Gnostic stream from its origin in Jewish heterodoxy towards its ending in Manichaeism. A new world religion comes to light.

The phenomenological school, more sceptical in its derivations and more respectful of facts, thinks it has a better conception of the historical evolution of Gnosticism than former generations had. But it also holds strongly that this religion has a sense in itself, which can be distinguished from other types of religion. Gnosis is always a knowledge of transcendent revelation, which makes the spiritual man aware of his real Self that is sleeping unconsciously in him, of its transcendent origin and ultimate destiny. This revelation has the form of a myth, not as a disguise of some philosophical abstractions, but because the myth is the spontaneous and adequate self-expression of the Gnostic soul. Therefore this myth should be read as a poem of religious experience, a divine comedy of longing and grace, which interprets the Universe as a mirror of inner moods. Earth arises from the state of despair, water from the tears of sorrow, air from the solidification of fear, light from laughter; while fire, causing death and destruction, is inherent in all these elements, as ignorance lies at the root of the other passions. Gnosis is the myth of the Self. So the phenomenological school seems to offer a picture of Gnosis which from an historical point of view is less improbable than the ill-founded hypotheses of the *Religionsgeschichtliche Schule* and does justice to the inner sense of this religious movement. Gnosticism, as far as it was important for the history of mankind, started among the heretical circles, the Minim of palestinian Judaism; it is a myth strongly rooted in a certain psychological attitude, in which the relation of man to himself, the world, and God is expressed. How was this relationship conceived?

What was the relation of the Gnostic to this world, in which he had to work and live? The new documents show us in a striking manner how the Gnostic experienced this world as complete nonsense, a bad dream and a cheap illusion—the world is an illusion. This is stated by the author of the 'Letter to Rheginos' in the following way; 'When you read in the Gospel that Elias and Moses appeared (on the occasion of the Transfiguration of Jesus on the mountain), you should not think that the resurrection is an illusion. Much more it should be said that the world—the cosmos—is an illusion: the living will die, the rich will become poor, everything changes, the world is an illusion.'

This conception recalls Indian speculations about the world as a veil of Maya. But the comparison should not seduce us immediately into supposing that these ideas were borrowed from Indian sources. The historical links, which may or may not exist, do not explain how it could happen that men of the second century B.C. had such a gloomy conception of the universe. The Greek philosophers of the time still sang their hymns in praise of that precious jewel which was the cosmos. The second century B.C. was a happy, prosperous, peaceful era, perhaps the happiest time that mankind ever knew. And yet these men, these Gnostics, conceived the world as an illusion, not because they borrowed this idea from India, but because they experienced the world as such.

The Gospel of Truth contains a wonderful passage about the world as a bad dream. It is unique in ancient literature and can have been written only by a poetical genius, as Valentinus was. It describes the state of ignorance, inconsistent illusion and absurdity, to which man in this world is condemned. 'Having no root, he thinks of himself: "I am like the shadows and the phantoms of the night". But when the light appears, he becomes aware that the fear which possessed him was nothing. So men were in ignorance of God, whom they did not see. When this ignorance created fear and trouble, made them uncertain, hesitating, divided and split, there were many vain illusions and empty and absurd fictions that vexed them, like dreamers in the grip of nightmares. You fly and do not know where, or you remain immovable when you are persecuting an unknown. You are fighting, give blows, receive blows. Or you fall from a height, or you fly in the air without wings. Sometimes it is as if you were killed by an invisible murderer, though you are not persecuted by anybody. Or it is as if you killed your neighbours, your hands are stained with blood. Till the moment that those who have gone through all these things, awake. Then they see nothing—those who have gone through all this—because these dreams were nothing. So they have thrown from them ignorance just as the dream that they also hold for nothing. And neither do they consider its works as realities, but they dismiss them as a nightmare.'

Valentinus expresses here, what so many poets before and after him have stated, that life in ignorance is a dream.

> Life's but a walking shadow, a poor player
> that struts and frets his hour upon the stage
> and then is heard no more: it is a tale
> told by an idiot, full of sound and fury
> signifying nothing.

I think we may state that the Gnostic has no relation to the world. He is living in a possessed world and he knows it. Now, of course, this conception of the world sounds very strange to progressive people who know so much and are so perfectly convinced of progress and the power of reason. We may, however, ask, which approach to reality happens to catch the essence of being, the rational approach or the existential, which necessarily expresses itself in myth. The other day I re-read that wonderful novel of Dostoevsky *The Possessed* in which he describes the first beginnings of the movement which is now in power in Russia. He describes it as a contagious state of possession and demonic insanity. How different is this picture from that which Turgenev drew, with great sympathy for revolutionary youth, in his *Fathers and Sons*. But history has shown that *Dostoevsky*'s outlook can be held with as good reasons as that of Turgenev. When the great Dutch historian Huizinga reviews the situation of modern man in the modern world, he begins his work, 'Shadows of Things to Come', with the words: 'We live in a possessed world and we know it'. This is pure mythology, and Huizinga knew it. But we cannot dismiss mythology when we want to express the essence of our being in the world. The rational approach to reality will always seem superficial and the existential approach fantastic. But both have their rights and it may be said that Valentinus, with the wonderful intuition of a poetic genius, expressed so many years ago what our tortured generation considers as its last word: that man in confronted with nothing.

We now proceed to discuss the relation of the Gnostic to God. Living in the world, in his state of ignorance, the Gnostic does not know that there is a God. The God of the Gnostic is the unknown God, infinitely removed from this unhappy world and its bloody history, and so also from man. The unknown God is so completely transcendent that he cannot be predicated, not even as being. Some Gnostics daringly spoke about the non-being God, the no-thing, beyond thinking and conscience and thought. And yet this unknown, this transcendent mystery, exercised a curious spell upon the Gnostic's mind. When God is absolutely unknown and unknowable, why should you speak about him? And yet the Gnostics were extremely eloquent when they had to express the idea in purely negative terms, that God is Depth and Silence. There was, according to them, an innate longing and craving in man to have relation with this transcendent mystery. And those who had received the grace to speak about that unknown Source of all being, which contains the Universe and is not contained by it, spoke with joy unspeakable about this bliss unspeakable:

'Not only he is what is called without beginning and without end, because he is ungenerated and immortal, but as he is without beginning and without end, so in his manner of being he is also unseizable in his greatness, unfathomable in his wisdom, unununderstandable in his power, impenetrable in his sweetness . . .'

'For, in fact, he is of such manner and immense greatness, that nothing else was with him from the beginning, no place wherein he dwells or whence he comes or whither he returns, no archetype which he uses as an image for his work, no trouble which accompanies him in his action, no underlying matter when he creates the things which he creates, no substance within him from which he produces the things which he produces, so that he could be accused of ignorance.'

'But as to himself, as he is and as he existeth and according to his manner of being, it is not possible that the intelligence knows him, nor that a word is capable of expressing him, nor that he can be seen or traced, owing to his unfathomable greatness and incomprehensible depth and immeasurable height and his unseizable will . . .'

'He is unknowable, that is, unthinkable by any thought, invisible in any way, unspeakable by any word, untouchable by any hand: he is the only one to know himself.'

These quotations, taken from the Treatise on the three natures, show convincingly what the Gnostics meant when they spoke about the unknown God. God is infinitely far above; man is on the earth, where he does not belong, a prey to possession and in complete ignorance of his transcendent origin and destination.

This complete lack of relationship is restored by the revelation of the Gnosis, mediated by the Saviour, who is Christ.

The Gospel of Truth contains a wonderful passage about the appeal to man by Christ, which makes him aware of his transcendent origin and ultimate destiny. Man, it seems, is conceived as a mountaineer who has lost his way and is wandering in the fog. Then he hears his name called; he knows where he came from and where he has to go to find his way back. This passage is perhaps the most characteristic of Gnosticism and clearly shows that Valentinus was both a poetic and a religious genius.

The Living Ones—that is to say, the Gnostics, whose names have been written in the Book of Life—receive their instruction for themselves alone. They turn to God in whom is the perfection of All, because they are those of whom the Father has known the names from the beginning and who are called at the end as beings who know that it is they whose names the Father has called. 'Therefore he who knows is a being from above. When he is called, he hears, he answers, he turns himself towards him who calls him. He comes to him, he understands how he has been called. Having the Gnosis, he fulfils the will of him that has called him and wants to do what pleases him. He receives rest. He who thus has the Gnosis, knows whence he comes and whither he goes; he understands as a man who has been drunk and awakens from the drunkenness wherein he was and comes to himself.' The Word of Christ is an event, an appeal which uncovers our deepest and innermost being; reminds it of its noble origin and glorious destiny, delivers it from the nightmares which it has produced by its unconsciousness and makes it aware of its unworldly essence. So through the appeal of the Saviour, which finds an echo in the spiritual man, the relation to God has been restored, and also the relation with the True Self, that divine spark of spirit which dreams unconsciously in man. Christ, for Valentinus, is the Word of God, which reveals man to himself.

It is this discovery of the unconscious Self which really matters in Gnosis. The whole religion can be summed up in the words of a Valentinian: 'The spirit, having become conscious of its origin, returned to its origin.' The complicated systems of Valentinus and Basilides in the second century, of Mani in the third century, are rooted in this basic experience. And the Gospel of Truth shows that this experience can be expressed even without a complicated system, which is still absent from this early writing. I think the new discovery plainly confirms the conception that the Gnostic myth is a projection, or, perhaps better, an expression of an emotional and overwhelming, irrational religious experience, the experience of the Self.

Thus man has gained, through revelation, a relation to himself and so to the unknown God. But what is the relation to his neighbour? What are the ethical implications of this religion? It is a very striking feature that in the Gospel of Truth ethical teaching is completely lacking. No commandments, no ethical considerations, nothing. Of course, it is very possible that Valentinus was a decent man, who behaved according to the rules of Christian or pagan morals. But Gnosis as such does not have ethical implications. It even seems that as often as not the Gnosics despised a proper behaviour according to the teaching of the Bible. They divided mankind into three classes which were different by nature: (1) the materialists, who were very bad and would perish without exception; (2) the psychics, the ordinary churchgoers, who had to do good works to be in their way; and (3) the spirited men who will be safe in any event, saved by nature, as they say. And, of course, the Gnostics belonged to those happy few who, far from the madding crowd, delighted in esoteric knowledge about the higher worlds and were too exalted to care about social obligations and social duties. Sometimes they taught a double morality; one for the mob, which is identical with the teaching of the church; and one for the Gnostics, which dismissed all categorical imperatives and looked on the world and the neighbour merely as means of self-realization.

In view of this, it is time to recall the distinction made by the Fathers of the Church, as well as by the apostles, between falsely so-called Gnosis and true Gnosis. Of course, these Fathers had perfectly good reason for rejecting the heretical Gnosis of their time; but at the same time they tried, with some success, to integrate the precious moments of this Gnosis into their own conception of Christianity. Clement of Alexandria and Origen claimed against Valentinus that they were the true Gnostics. Perhaps the theological disputes of that time are no longer relevant to modern man. But the problem as such still exists and can be put in modern terms. The false Gnosis does not know the encounter with another person. It considers man as an atom without windows, which must develop itself at all costs. Imagine those old gentlemen, those dear ladies, who are so entirely concentrated on their divine self. Even intercourse with women becomes a means of self-realization: it enables man to experience his transcendent, hermaphroditic unity. As a matter of fact this was what the Valentinians of the second century taught. Then, however, man does not meet another being, whose other-ness he respects, but uses his neighbour as an instrument. That is the false Gnosis. To Gnostics of this kind the apostle Paul says: 'If somebody imagines that he has Gnosis, he has not yet learned to know as he ought to know.'

When then is true Gnosis? From the Christian point of view, true Gnosis considers the encounter with the neighbour as a religious experience. There exists a wonderful saying of Jesus, not contained in our Gospels, which nevertheless may be authentic: 'Have you seen your brother, you have seen your Lord'. The neighbour is a mysterious other, who comes on our way and represents the Lord. The poor, the miserable, the sick, the doomed should be seen, really seen, because behind them, in solidarity with them, is the suffering servant.

Of course, the Gnostics were and are right in their criticism of current Christian morals. The Christian faith, however, is not a credulous acceptance of what the Church says or the Bible says, but is the personal encounter with Christ. Those who have some insight into the person of Jesus affirm that this encounter must have, and cannot but have, ethical implications. The consequence of this encounter might be that man becomes one with the mob, the condemned, or even humiliates himself so far as to range himself among the ordinary church-goers.

And this encounter will certainly change his attitude towards the world and its suffering. For Paul, the Gnosis of Christ implied the voluntary acceptance of world suffering: 'If we know Christ and the communion with his suffering and the force of his resurrection.' The false Gnostic rejects martyrdom; the true Gnostic accepts martyrdom. Origen died in consequence of the wounds inflicted on him during persecutions by the State. Now imagine a spiritual leader who tried to persuade his fellow-religionists not to resist the totalitarian State. Would not he be, for all his spiritual insight, a false gnostic? So we may imagine that the Christian Church, even of our time, would reject a Gnosis which considers man as a spiritual atom without windows, a self-realizing individual lacking relationship with his neighbours. But the judgement of the Fathers was not only negative. Some of them knew perfectly well how unspiritual the mass of Christians can be, and how unsatisfactory for the religious temperament the answers of the official Church sometimes are. That is why they presented their teaching as the true Gnosis. For Gnosis it remained. And it is most appealing for a modern mind to see how practically all the fathers of the Church, not only Origen but also St. Augustine, speak about the 'Gnosis' of the self. They have integrated this conception in the whole of their teaching. According to them, knowledge of your self is a stage on the way to knowledge of God!

Were they right? Is it Christian to speak about love for your self, as for instance St. Augustine does? The great commandment, the corollary of the Christian religion is to love God and your neighbours as yourself. This, it seems, does imply that man loves himself. It is shown to him how he will be a proper man, an *imago Dei*, when he answers to the Calling of Christ, the Word of God, and so encounters his neighbour. Then he really is himself in his relationship to the other. Then he really loves himself. Therefore, I think, the Fathers of the Church were quite right when they considered the Gnosis of the Self as part of the Christian religion. It is perhaps a merit of the heretical Gnostics that they drew the attention of their contemporaries to this unconscious Self that is sleeping in man.

Economics and the Individual

S. ADLER

Department of Applied Economics, Cambridge

ECONOMICS IS, of course, the study of economic interrelations, or, as Alfred Marshall defined it with deliberate looseness, the study of mankind in the ordinary business of life. It is generally regarded with envy by other social scientists because the interrelations with which it deals are frequently quantifiable and because their structure can sometimes be expressed in terms of systems of interdependent functions. But while they can be described in terms of more and less, they are not always measurable. Even when they are, they tend to be so less accurately and more conditionally than is the case with the interrelations studied by the natural sciences, where measurement lends itself to the formulation of specific operational instructions. Broadly speaking, in natural science there are usually some invariants, whereas in economics there are not—that is from the point of view of measurement. This is not to deny that economics is perhaps more advanced than the other social sciences, or that it is so because its subject-matter lends itself, however roughly, to quantification.

There is space here to consider only a few broad aspects of economic interrelations. First, it is necessary to emphasize that economics is a *social* science and therefore deals with *social* interrelations. It is not the investigation of the pure logic of choice in a vacuum, or of individual economic activity in isolation. Nothing shows this more conclusively than the fact that the Robinson Crusoe of the primers is never an isolated individual—except physically—but a man who carries his society and its values, or rather the society and values of the primer writer, with him. Economists, no matter how bloodless their categories or impalpable their abstractions, must postulate some social and institutional framework for economic behaviour. Economic interrelations are through and through social, they are relations between persons or between groups of persons in society. And one must never forget this elementary fact.

It is precisely because these interrelations are social that economic invariants are so elusive, if not impossible to find. For the same reason, economic interrelations are not always quantifiable, and when quantifiable not always measurable, and when measurable often only conditionally and, so to speak, in quotation marks. It is for this same reason that the mathemactical theory of games, a branch of mathematics created by Von Neumann and dealing with strategies in zero sum games, is largely of peripheral interest to economists[1]. It may shed some light on the strategies adopted by oligopolists, a small number of sellers dominating a market, or by oligopsonists, a small number of buyers dominating a market. But, at any rate in its present form, it does not seem applicable on an extensive scale to *la condition économique humaine*, which is incapable of reduction to a zero sum game or to any concatenation of zero sum games.

There is a second aspect of economic interrelations to which I wish to refer. Historically, they have become both more integrated and more complex in the course of time. In the most

[1]Zero sum games are games in which the loser's, or losers', losses exactly equal the winner's, or winners', gains. Poker is clearly a zero sum game. Speculation on the stock market is already less simple, especially in periods of rising or falling prices, unless, that is, one widens the universe of discourse sufficiently. The *joie de jouer* in zero sum games is a complication the mathematician must abstract from; which is another illustration *in parvo* of the difficulties attendant upon quantification and measurement in economics. There is an interesting parallel between the genesis of the theory of probability and that of the theory of games. The former started from a question posed by a gambler to Pascal and Fermat, the latter from a consideration of optimal strategies in poker. No wonder that Von Neumann's and Morgenstern's *Mathematical Theory of Games and Economic Behaviour* has been described as the most sinister book since Machiavelli's *The Prince*,

primitive self-sufficient economy, where there is direct consumption of what is directly produced by the same person or same small group of persons, they are relatively simple. In the still primitive but more advanced economy, in which a large part of economic activity does not centre on the market but in which there is some exchange, they are already more complex. Money may not yet be essential, if exchange is casual or intermittent and indulged in on a barter basis of goods against goods. But as production and wants expand, as exchange increases and becomes more routinized, money becomes more indispensable.

In a society such as our own, in which so much of production is indirect or roundabout, to use Böhm-Bawerk's term, and in which the greater part of economic behaviour becomes subsumable under market activity, economic interrelations are incomparably more complicated. Most economic activity now involves a wider and wider network of transactions with greater and greater ramifications. When transactions embracing broader groups and sub-groups of individuals, locally, regionally, nationally and internationally, are entered into, money is absolutely indispensable as a unit of account, a medium of exchange and a store of value.

When I buy tea, I am entering into economic relations with the tea planter of Assam or Ceylon; the shipper, who arranges for its delivery in London; the blender; the wholesaler, who arranges its distribution; the banker, who finances production or shipment or distribution, or all three; the retailer, who sells me the tea; not to mention the Governments, which tax the tea at the points of export or import[1]. The tea planter must employ labour, purchase or hire land, and buy machinery, fertilisers, etc., from various manufacturers and merchants. My demand for tea depends on the demand of all other tea consumers. It also depends on my demand for other beverages, which in turn depends on my demand for other commodities and groups of commodities. In technical parlance, it is an item in my scale of preferences, which is affected by everyone else's scale of preferences.

[1]The British tax on tea takes the form of an excise tax and not of a tariff or import duty. But the net effect is substantially the same.

Indirectly, therefore, when I buy tea, I am entering into economic relations with all the parties concerned in the production and consumption of tea; and, in the last analysis, I am also entering into economic relations with the people participating in the production and consumption of every other commodity produced and marketed on a significant scale. These relations are of varying degrees of propinquity and distance, and the constellations it is necessary to analyse depend on the appropriate level of scientific abstraction. In practice, I am usually conscious only of my direct relation with the retailer and am unaware of, or forget, the innumerable other relations involved. Consequently, when I find the market price of tea too high, I tend to make the retailer the scapegoat. But my lack of awareness or obliviousness of these relations does not affect their existence.

In no society, however advanced, does the market become all-embracing. When the housewife cooks and washes for her family, she is performing functions which, if performed by someone else, are remunerated approximately in accordance with the forces of the market-place. If I hire a domestic servant, the wages I pay her will be determined by the state of the labour market and by what she can get elsewhere in the same or a similar occupation. For the middle-class wife, at any rate, there is a very real range of choice between doing work outside the home and hiring domestic service, on the one hand, and foregoing outside work and doing her own housekeeping, on the other. But while a domestic servant's wages are included in the national income, a housewife's unremunerated services are not. Hence Pigou's paradox that the national income falls when a man marries his housekeeper.[1] However, if the market never becomes all-embracing, it does become more and more pervasive, so that non-market behaviour has

[1]This is the kind of problem, sometimes theoretical, sometimes practical, sometimes both, which so frequently crops up in economic measurement. The concept of the national income is fundamental in economics. Yet its measurement raises a hornet's nest of difficulties, some subtle and *raffiné*, others crude and blatant. This is one reason, among others, why economists treat the published data on the national income with many more reservations than do non-economists.

increasingly less *economic* significance. From which it does not follow that the *non*-economic significance of such behaviour also declines.

The emergence of wider regional and national markets and, indeed, of the world market was a condition precedent to the Industrial Revolution of the late eighteenth and nineteenth centuries. Large-scale factory production presupposes broad and expanding outlets for the absorption of the commodities it turns out. Adam Smith's saying, 'The division of labour is limited by the extent of the market,' is both platitudinous and profound. Platitudinous, because it is obvious at inspection; profound, because it illuminates many historical phenomena which are not so obvious, either at inspection or after close study. Thus, it is an integral part of the answer to the question why the rate of economic expansion in America has been greater than in Britain. It helps to explain why mass production and mass *consumption* are so closely linked. It also helps in understanding why our economic system, *qua* economic system, has reached its apogee in the United States, a country which is free of any vestigial traces of feudalism and, therefore, of any relics of a relatively static stratification of tastes as well as of rôles in the productive process. And, not least, it focuses attention on one of the crucial problems in the economic growth of backward and under-developed countries, namely the creation of a wide internal market. This problem is sometimes forgotten in the plethora of blueprints of Five-Year Plans concentrating on the expansion of industrial production in countries and areas, where market relations cover only a small part of economic activity.

Third, the path of evolution towards complex and integrated economic interrelations has not occurred uniformly or in a straight line. Purely in terms of abstract logic, one might think that no insulated or partially insulated local, regional or national markets would survive, and that the first would be completely embraced by or articulated in the second, the second by the third, and the third by a single omnivorous world market. Historically, this has not been the case. There is, of course, a very meaningful and highly pertinent sense in which we can talk of a world economy. No country is autarchic. Each country has economic interrelations with other countries. This is self-evident for the United Kingdom, which depends for its very existence as an advanced economy on its ability to export manufactured goods in payment for the food and raw materials it imports. But it is also true of the United States, which is much more richly endowed in natural resources. America not only needs external outlets for some of its manufactures and for its surplus agricultural products; it also needs external sources of supply for certain foodstuffs, raw materials, non-ferrous metals and even highly specialized manufactures.

There is room only for two or three examples of the discontinuous and staccato nature of economic development.

The first example derives from what men have *thought* about economic trends. The gospel of Free Trade envisaged an ultimate goal in which national markets were so loosely separated that they constituted, in effect, a single decompartmentalized world market. It arose and flourished in England in the nineteenth century. Retrospectively, it is easy to see why the ideology of Free Trade triumphed where and when it did—England had a head start in the world market. When the advantages attendant on a head start weakened or disappeared, so did the doctrine. It never enjoyed elsewhere the success and prestige it attained in England, because other countries were engaged in catching up, in developing their own domestic markets and in extending their share in the world market. Interestingly enough, it has tended to become orthodoxy in contemporary America, but on a less general scale and in a peculiarly attenuated form. American free trade—capital letters would be deceptive—envisages and claims a much greater degree of protection for the home market, with all the paraphernalia of technical Customs obstacles, escape clauses, gentleman's agreements, etc., than was ever the case with the British version in its heyday. The pure milk of the gospel has turned sour in its journey across the ocean and over the century.

The fact that backward countries were often partially integrated into the world market *before* they had evolved a genuine national or domestic market provides a second example of discontinuous development. This happened in Iran and China in the past and is happening today in the

Rhodesias and East and West Africa, where it is the more striking because they are the more backward. The process is fraught with grave consequences at an economic as at other levels for the countries and areas concerned, enhancing as it does the instability, and hence endangering the viability, of their social structures.

Finally, there are now two separate world markets, the market of the Soviet bloc and that of the rest of the world. These two markets though interrelated, since they trade with each other, are nevertheless distinct. One has only to look at the shift in the foreign trade of China, which previously conducted a negligible volume of trade with the Soviet bloc and now carries on roughly 80 per cent of its foreign commerce within the bloc, to realize that this point is of more than taxonomic interest.

In sum, there have always been conflicts between the centripetal and centrifugal tendencies in the economic process, and the balance between them is forever precarious and shifting. The theory of imperfect competition, one of the outstanding contributions of economic analysis in the last thirty years, is a powerful weapon in the understanding of the persistence and tenacity of the centrifugal tendencies in the face of the vigorous unfolding of the centripetal. It helps to elucidate both the growth of trusts and giant concerns and the survival of smaller-scale and even small-scale producers; both the expansion of multiple shops and department stores and the survival of the corner tobacconist and grocer. Competition is never perfect, nor monopoly pure, in real life. Competition is itself the mother of oligopoly and monopoly, and monopoly is itself unstable and competitive.

The last two aspects of economic interrelations I shall discuss are of immediate interest to psychologists, of whatever school. With the growth in the scale of production and the increasing subsumption of economic activity under the forces of the market, economic interrelations become depersonalized.[1] In what seventeenth and eighteenth century

[1]Depersonalization is the least obnoxious English translation of the German word *Verdinglichung*. The more affirmative translations of the sociologists, 'reification' and 'thingification', are literary monstrosities.

writers were pleased to call the state of nature, if ever such existed, economic relations were direct and personal. Even at as late a historical stage as feudalism, economic inter-relations were to a great extent determined by *direct* personal interrelations. But in our society relations between persons become mediated and indirect and begin to appear as relations between persons and things. In the example cited above I am largely unaware of my very real relations with the people in-volved in the production, distribution and consumption of tea. And what is true for me is also true for the other people con-cerned with tea. They are as little aware of their relations with me as I am of mine with them. As already indicated, this in no way detracts from the existence of such relations. Naturally, when things go wrong, as in an acute coal shortage or in a transportation strike, I become much more aware, however distinctly or indistinctly, of these interrelations. But with the resumption of normalcy, this awareness fades and is soon obliterated.

It is essential to add one vital qualification, a qualification which may itself be a signpost. In periods such as World War II, when the existence of the community as a whole is at stake, most people become conscious of a common and actively shared goal. The non-economic aspects of our economic inter-relations are much more prominent, and *pro tanto* the merely economic aspects tend to recede in importance. It is easier to see the social purpose of the things we are making and doing, and our interrelations consequently appear more immediate and direct. The producers of tanks and aeroplanes know *and feel* that they are tied to the ultimate users of the product by more than the cash nexus. To those who grow food, whether on the farm, in the garden or on the allotment, 'Food for Victory' is not an empty advertising slogan but a vivid expres-sion both of the communal will and of the cultivators' ability to contribute to its realization.

I am not implying that the identification of individual with social goals or the awareness of other human beings as ends and only ends are thoroughgoing even in wartime. The moratorium on selfishness is never complete, and any trans-formation of this kind is conditioned and limited by the background in which it occurs. It suffices for my argument that the individual is much more conscious than he usually is of active participation in a common purpose and that his day-to-day conduct is substantially influenced by this consciousness. The paradox that this temporary and partial resolution of the conflict between individual and social ends requires the stimulus of war for its achievement is too striking to call for extended comment. And, again, once the attainment of the common goal is assured, a marked relapse is liable to occur, although the experience of group solidarity survives in the mystic chords of memory.

Many people with a nostalgia for the past, as well as other critics of contemporary civilization, have eloquently bewailed this depersonalization. As relations between persons become ostensibly transformed into relations between persons and things, the human being, the personality itself, becomes a commodity, a means and not an end. Some relations which are highly personal in essence are distorted in a bizarre way. Art itself becomes a commodity.

To take an obvious example. The cinema is the specific art form of the twentieth century . It involves an advanced productive apparatus and an intricate market mechanism for its continued existence and is deeply enmeshed in the network of commodity relations. It is not surprising, therefore, that it is the most commercialized of all the arts. An actor as fresh and invigorating as was Barry Fitzgerald when he was with the Abbey Theatre suffers a sea change, not into something rich and strange, but into a standardized and mechanical collection of tricks when transposed to the cinema. His greatest assets generate equal and opposite liabilities when converted into box office appeal. The same thing is happening, albeit more slowly and unevenly, to the Italian cinema, which has produced the most stimulating and original of all post-war films partly because it was the most direct and least alienated in its handling of human beings.

The commercialization of the cinema is the outcome not only of the large-scale capital investment needed for producing and exhibiting films, but also of the separation of the participants in the making of a film from the consumer, which is another facet of depersonalization. The film producer's prime interest in the film audience is pecuniary. Sometimes it is his sole interest. In such circumstances art is at best a by-product of the elaborate movie industry, and it is a wonder not that so many bad films are produced but that some good ones are produced at all.

What holds for the cinema also holds, if not as crudely or to the same extent, for the other arts. However ivory his tower or Dionysiac his urge, the artist must function within the framework, economically speaking, of a 'rationally calculating society'. As art becomes a commodity, success breeds failure as its almost inevitable reward.

Depersonalization is so noticeable in art because of the intensely personal nature of the acts of creation and response, the patent confusion of means and ends and the irrelevance of the values of the market-place. But it is present, at least as much if not more, in other fields where pecuniary values are more easily taken for granted. To venture on perhaps too simple a generalization, the degree of depersonalization in any particular sphere of economic activity tends to vary inversely with the importance of the non-economic content or of the non-economic aspects of the interrelations concerned. Since in the nature of the case economic interrelations have non-economic aspects, and since the lines of demarcation between the economic and non-economic are anything but clear, there is an inevitable blurring of the edges between means and ends.

When we witness a particularly flagrant treatment of human beings as means and only means, our conscience, our sense of decency, revolts. But the conscience has its economy too. We cannot forever be thinking too precisely on the event. Life is too short for us to be continually unravelling the knots of our economic interrelations, or every transaction, however commonplace, would demand an inordinate mental effort. And, in the last analysis, it is not merely a matter of our individual mental and moral limitations, as Tolstoy supposed. We can no more escape society than we can escape history.

The conscience also has its quirks. There are few indeed who will not strain at gnats to swallow camels. Human beings combine hypersensitivity on some issues with anaesthesia on others.

The most explosive and banal, although by no means narrowly economic, contemporary example of depersonalization is to be found in the fate of the nuclear physicist. He is our latter-day *Zauberlehrling*, both out of control of and 'dissociated' from what he has conjured up. Here depersonalization borders perilously close on complete alienation, with dire consequences for himself no less than for the community of which he is a member.

The concept we are discussing may sound a remote and nebulous abstraction. But if carried far enough in its concrete manifestations, it begins to mean ceasing to treat others as human beings and, therefore, ceasing to be a human being oneself. In Kant's classic formulation, human beings constitute the kingdom of ends. Where depersonalization is untrammelled, it entails *dehumanization*. Human beings become means and only means, and not the perverse mixtures, so impervious to analysis, of means and ends we remain to each other. Our generation has already once suffered the terrible scourge of dehumanization on a massive scale. Let not this scourge be dismissed as exclusively or predominantly an individual madman's handiwork. We should likewise beware of explaining it—or rather, explaining it away—as the consequence of destructive demonic tendencies latent or present in all, including the best, of us. It is seriously suggested that the depersonalization pervading our economic interrelations may be one element, and an important one at that, in a more adequate account of Nazism, a movement which has not yet been definitively dissected in all its many-sided socio-pathological implications.

It goes without saying that there is another side to the medal, a side too familiar to require more than cursory mention. Depersonalization has been the inevitable concomitant of greater economic integration and complexity. This complexity has yielded an enormously heightened mastery over nature, an incomparable expansion of productive capacity, a manifold increase both in our command over goods and services and in the accessibility of non-material values to the vast majority of the population of the industrialized countries, at any rate. The poorest member of our community is richer in these respects than the African king, who—to quote Adam Smith's celebrated apostrophe—was 'the absolute master of the lives and liberties of ten thousand naked savages.' In short, modern society, for good as well as for ill, would be unthinkable without a highly evolved and advanced pattern of economic interrelations.

In terms of personal relations, the routinization of transactions associated with rational economic calculation is much less cumbersome, much more time- and energy-saving, than all previous alternatives. The marked contrast with the personal entanglements encountered in economic activity in feudal or caste society, for instance, is indubitably to our advantage. After all, when I want to buy something, I *generally* do not want to consider all the nuances of my attitude to the seller and of his to me, not to mention the other people connected with its manufacture and distribution. I do not want to engage in that endless battle of wits so often waged over even the simplest transaction in pre-modern markets, to which the application of the mathematical theory of games might be so apt were it not for the participants' manifest pleasure in the contest as such. To us it is an added advantage, to be taken as a matter of course, that so many of our purchases are of standardized goods at uniform prices, and that so many of our transactions are consummated in the twinkling of an eye. Such a *modus operandi* would be repugnant if not undignified in a bazaar. We prefer to play most of our games in other fashions, although there is a definite game element in certain economic activities and interrelations in our society too. But this is not the place to compile a balance sheet, if that is *la phrase juste*.

To repeat, the increasing rationalization of economic activity and of economic calculation is accompanied by increasing depersonalization. Now the essence of rational economic calculation consists in its being an admirable instrument for dealing with means. For this very reason, at a certain point *rational economic calculation becomes irrational*. Rationality about means becomes irrationality about ends precisely because some means are also ends and some ends also means. The kingdom of ends and the republic of means are not separate territories, with a readily ascertainable boundary between them. But the rational and irrational do not fuse. They conjoin in a schizophrenic syncretism which lies at the heart of the paradox of reason in unreason and of unreason in reason. The artist's dilemma of failure in success is but one instance of this paradox. We are all familiar with it at divers levels, sometimes more trivial, sometimes more profound. It is the subject, or at any rate the point, of countless jokes of the *New Yorker* cartoon genre as well as the source of the humour and pathos of, say, Chaplin's *Modern Times*, which I like to think will be prescribed 'seeing' for students of history and the social sciences a hundred years hence.

These considerations lead directly to my conclusion. Rational economic calculation goes with pecuniary calculation or valuation. And, in turn, our pecuniary values are an essential ingredient, nay, part of the core of our general scheme of values. Thorstein Veblen, perhaps the most distinguished social scientist the United States has produced, attempted to elaborate a social theory in which the distinction between the pecuniary and the industrial, between making money and making things, plays a large part. This distinction is not unilluminating and seems to have constituted the starting point of some of his most original and brilliant insights.[1] He especially emphasized the conflicts between 'the instinct of workmanship' and the pecuniary drive. His views on the historical and doctrinal connexions between the emergence of economic theory as the analysis of rational economic calculation and the acceptance, perhaps implicit at least as much as explicit, of natural rights, natural law and utilitarianism have largely been ignored. It may, however, be of some interest that Myrdal, starting from very different economic and philosophic preconceptions, reaches similar conclusions, at any rate in so far as the historical

[1]Veblen is best known in this country for his *Theory of the Leisure Class*, a number of phrases from which, such as 'conspicuous consumption' and 'conspicuous waste', have entered the language. It is to be regretted that some of his other works are not more widely read. In my opinion, his *Imperial Germany and the Industrial Revolution*, which was first published forty years ago, still remains one of the best single books on Germany. It enjoyed the odd distinction of having been simultaneously barred from the mails by one branch of the United States Government and used as propaganda against the enemy by another during World War I.

connexions between economic theory and natural law are concerned.[1] Veblen did not succeed in forming an influential school, and none of his professed followers have proved themselves capable of duplicating his *aperçus*.

The problem of ranking pecuniary values in the general hierarchy of values, whether social or individual, clearly transcends any single intellectual discipline and belongs, perhaps, to the discredited realm of metaphysics. It would be out of order to flounder in such deep if not imaginary waters. I wish, however, to cite an historical phenomenon which may be of some pertinence to the psychologist, and, more specifically, to the social psychologist. A hyperinflation can be loosely described as an inflation in which the purchasing power of money virtually vanishes. Very few inflations, fortunately, degenerate into hyperinflations. The fall in the purchasing power of money in an inflation may be sustained and sharp, as in England during World Wars I and II, for instance, but it is not catastrophic as in a hyperinflation such as occurred in Germany in the aftermath of its defeat in World War I. In other words, a hyperinflation is an inflation which has got out of hand.

Now in all hyperinflations of which we have record pecuniary values become grossly distorted. In comparatively normal situations, the relations between the prices of different commodities are fairly stable and form a pattern which we accept as standard or customary. Not so in hyperinflation. The conventional price relationships break down, and their pattern becomes crazy. Our pecuniary scales are corroded and eventually collapse.[2] With this corrosion of the structure of pecuni-

[1]See Myrdal, *The Political Element in the Development of Economic Theory*, (Routledge and Kegan Paul) London, 1953. The new Preface to the English edition contains a most stimulating and candid discussion of the inescapability of value assumptions in *any* economic theorizing, however formal. Myrdal's discussion is the more impressive because it would appear to be partly the result of his reflections on his own productive labours in sociology and administration.

[2]It may be worth adding that the first function of money to be impaired and eventually shattered in hyperinflation is the most advanced, namely, its function as a store of value, and the last the most elementary, namely, its function as a unit of account; naturally, there is simultaneity and overlapping here too.

ary values the corrosion of the traditional order or structure of ethical values follows suit.

This temporal sequence (in any case, this is a simplification, since there is a considerable degree of synchronization) does not necessarily imply causal sequence. It may be that the corrosion of pecuniary values is an effect rather than a cause, or, more plausibly, as much an effect as a cause, of the corrosion of other values. But, whatever the causal priorities, what does emerge from the course of events in hyperinflations is that pecuniary values appear to pervade and suffuse the hierarchy of values as a whole. The nexus of values is interacting and reciprocal. When one group of values is damaged, so are the others. If it is objected that this interaction occurs only in periods of acute strain and stress, one need only compare our society with primitive or less developed societies to see that this interconnexion is not uniquely confined to hyperinflation. Even in periods of inflation, there is a general weakening of the fabric of values, manifested in Britain, for example, by the growth of spivs and under-the-counter dealings as well as by the statistics of crime and juvenile delinquency; this weakening occurs on a much smaller and less dramatic scale, but it is there all the same. What distinguishes hyperinflation in this respect is that the interconnexion between pecuniary and other values becomes more starkly apparent.

There is an important corollary to the thesis that pecuniary values pervade the hierarchy of values. The more a society is characterized by rational economic calculation and, which comes to the same thing, by the predominance of economic activity with reference to a market, the greater the extent to which pecuniary valuation pervades the pattern of values as a whole. Or, to put it negatively, the general pattern of values in such a society is more vulnerable to a collapse of pecuniary values. The German hyperinflation after World War I and the Chinese during and after World War II form an instructive contrast in this respect. Because China was less urbanized, less industrialized and less economically integrated than Germany, the Chinese hyperinflation was much less disastrous in its impact on accepted norms of conduct *in general* than was the German. Even the Chinese middle-class, which was much smaller proportionately, was far less demoralized—in the literal sense—than was the German.[1] It is, of course, to be expected that greater economic complexity entails greater economic vulnerability. Perhaps it should not be so surprising that it entails greater vulnerability in other spheres of behaviour than the economic. A suggestion worthy of consideration is that the degree of stress on and corrosion of general values in periods of economic cataclysm is related to the degree of depersonalization in a given society.

The general and particular ills attendant on depersonalization lend themselves more readily to diagnosis than to prescription and cure. One significant if trite conclusion to be derived from our diagnosis is that concentrating on the individual in abstraction from society is as one-sided as concentrating on society in abstraction from the individual. Society and the individuals constituting society are correlative. The individual is as much a product of society as society is of the individual. It is dangerous, therefore, to endeavour to treat either of the correlatives in separation from the other. The resolution of the dilemma of reason in unreason or of unreason in reason is to be sought, if sought at all, by individuals at a social level.

[1]The demoralization of the German middle class in the hyperinflation undoubtedly facilitated the rise of Nazism.

Man and the Machine

JOHN A. MACK

Stevenson Lecturer in Citizenship, University of Glasgow

I SHALL TAKE a pretty wide cast. I want first to refer to the unproductivity of productivity campaigns. Then I propose to examine the problem of Job. Not the problem of the job, as the context might suggest; but the problem of Job, the book in the Old Testament. Then I shall discuss the importance of not discussing the human factor in industry, or 'The Dangers of being Articulately Human'. Then I want to consider the anthropologist in his rôle of philosophical smuggler, or the surreptitious importation of value judgements; then I shall go on to the subject of '*Woman* and the Machine' which is going to be a bigger problem in the future than the subject of this chapter. I can hardly cover all that ground; but these are my intentions.

In talking about human relations in industry there is usually an unexpressed premiss; that if one looks after the human relations in industry, if one pays special attention to the human or non-technical organization in factories, coal mines and so on, it will follow as the night the day that production will go up. I suggest that this premiss is of doubtful validity. It is quite possible to attend very carefully to the human relations in industry, and as a result have production go down. The whip might get more production than the carrot even over long periods. It has happened. There are examples of it. At least (to sum up) one should not assume that the humanization of industry will make for greater productivity. Why not? Because generally speaking (I suggest) the spirit in which most managers study human relations in industry is wrong. They have their eye all the time on the main chance; they make the same mistake as was made by Job.

May I refer you now to 'Studies in the Philosophy of Religion', by Archibald Allan Bowman? I think it is one of the best treatments of the problem of Job and of the Old Testament. Most of the books in the Old Testament have the healthy belief that if you behave well, then you will be duly rewarded towards the end of the day or even before.

> And thou shall do that which is right and good in the sight of the Lord that it may be well with thee: that thou mayest go in and possess the land which the good Lord sweareth unto thy fathers.

In other words, do good and right in the sight of the Lord and He will reward you. And if you want to know in what sense, there it is—'that thou mayest go in and possess the land which the Lord sweareth unto thy fathers'. The Good Earth here and now. That is, I think, fairly generally agreed to be the morality of the Old Testament. Do what you ought to do, worship as you ought to worship, work as you ought to work, and you will get your reward here and now.

Job, if you remember, is a problem to himself, and to his advisers, and to students of the Old Testament, because he seemed in every respect to do all that was required of him, and still everything happened to him which shouldn't have happened. But the New Testament resolves the problem. Some of its most famous sayings seem to repeat the Old Testament. I have never forgotten John MacMurray on that famous Beatitude, Blessed are the Meek. Why are the meek blessed? *For they shall inherit the earth.* MacMurray points out that we all remember the first bit, 'Blessed are the Meek'. It is a good thing to believe. But we never take seriously the sequel, 'For they shall inherit the earth'. MacMurray, of course, takes it quite seriously. 'Blessed are the meek, for they *shall* inherit the earth', he says. Now does not this justify Job's laments? No. The whole point is that if you are out to inherit the earth, you cannot be really meek. A meek person is someone who never thinks about inheriting the earth. He will inherit the earth because he is truly meek. And so I go on to that ultimate message which says 'Seek ye first the Kingdom of God and . . .'

That is the trouble about modern industry. Industrial managers seek first more productivity, and they are going to treat their workers as human beings—a thing they do not appear to have done before—because that is the way to get more productivity. Hence the paradox of productivity over the past fifty years, particularly in the mines. Up till very recently, the great influx of mechanical methods of coal winning, particularly of coal cutting and coal conveying, has not increased the output per man in the pits over fifty years; or has increased it only very slightly and that in recent years. Over the period as a whole we still have the remarkable phenomenon that mechanization, introduced so as to secure a substantial increase in output per man-hour, simply has not done it. Of course, there are all manner of technical reasons for this failure. Coal is a wasting asset: it keeps on getting further away from the shaft: and so on. But still there is a problem here.

And then we have the working parties going to America and coming back with all manner of notions about how to improve productivity. Slight improvements are being made all over the place; they would have to be with all that effort; but nothing like what they should be. Because, people say, to improve productivity we must change the attitude of our workers, and that means changing the attitude of managements. That is to say, we must create better human relations in industry so as to get more productivity. Naturally, they don't get more productivity. If only they would read Job intelligently!

The great new steel plants are encountering strange and unexpected things. Coal firing was, not exactly dangerous, but a very dirty and heavy job for the furnace men. Fired by oil, the job becomes relatively simple. You go over and turn the tap on, and go over later and turn the tap off. The change was made in one particular establishment. The furnace workers were given the new job of oil firing and of turning the tap on and off. They looked at the new set-up, it was nice and shiny—

and turned to each other saying, 'No, it won't do'. 'We'll claim walking money', they said. 'We'll claim walking money'. And so they sat down and wouldn't do another stroke until they were paid for walking over and turning the tap on, and walking back later and turning the tap off.

Now, they were being given a much nicer job, a much cleaner job, a much healthier job, and quite as well paid. But they wanted walking money for the walking part of it. Another example is from another famous plant. Nowadays the steel is cut into strips entirely by a mechanical process. The people who control this process do so from a travelling crane well above the floor. The strips of steel move along down below, about the height of this roof from this floor. The worker sits in his chair, moving a lever back and forward. The former method was a desperately hot business, the all but molten steel moving along and the men actually cutting it into bars with great shears. It was a very hot and a very uncomfortable job. The men sweated profusely. They actually bit on dirty rags, the heat was so overpowering. And now they are sitting in a chair away up there, moving the lever. And they like it, mind you. But a claim was recently made from the chap sitting up in the chair for heat money, because at that infinitesimal point of time when the hot strips came below his bottom, he felt the slight heat. That was uncomfortable—so he claimed heat money.

My third example is from the coal mines. It is an old example: it is about four or five years old.

In a particular pit in Scotland they had actually brought daylight into the face. Normally in any coal mine it is very dark underground. But in some collieries where the atmosphere permits, where there isn't much in the way of gas, they can have electric or other forms of lighting brought to the face; and they brought fluorescent lighting to this particular face. The men were now able to see clearly what they had been doing. On this particular face, the roof was a good height, about twelve feet high. Miners build up wooden packs, as they call them, wooden baulks, criss-crossed, to hold the roof up. The colliers looked around when the lighting came on the face and saw the wooden packs they had been building. And they saw how big they were—'Big as a bloody house, man'—they said to each other. Big as a house, and all for the ordinary money! So as soon as they saw the height of this house they had been building, they sat down and wouldn't do another stroke until they got five shillings a shift more.

Workers are ungrateful people. Is that the moral? In all three cases the conditions had been enormously improved from your point of view and my point of view. Conditions are much more *human*. And what is the reaction of these trade-unionists and workers? They at once begin to say, 'How can we make more money out of these people?' I don't know how the first two cases come out, but I know how the third one came out. They sat there for three days, let's say from Monday to Wednesday, and the Manager didn't normally come round that part of the big pit until Thursday, so he didn't know officially they were sitting down. He knew perfectly well. He knew five minutes after they started. But he didn't know officially. So he came round on the Thursday in the normal manner and he saw these men sitting there and of course he was much surprised. He said, 'Why are you sitting there, gentlemen?'—or words to that effect—and they explained to him why they were sitting there, and he explained to them how really conditions were so much better than before, since they could now see what they were doing, and they said, Well, now that they could see what they were doing, they could see how they had been fooled in the past and he was lucky that they weren't claiming a retrospective price of five shillings per shift for the previous ten or twenty or fifty years! Finally the Manager conceded half a crown more on the shift. And ever after that he was known in the district as Santa Claus.

That was the reaction of the mining specialists. Mining engineers know exactly what they want to do; they know exactly how the men should behave and are thoroughly shocked when the men don't behave as expected. They have the mechanical side taped, they have the supplies and materials taped, they have the machines taped; all they have to tape now is the human factor, and they go on to tape that; and then they are very much surprised when the output per man shift throughout the country remains round about the same level.

I have put this particular case, which is a good test-case, to different groups of colliery managers. I have asked them, 'Now, was this the action of a good manager or a bad manager?' and they all said he was a bad manager to have given way. So I put it to them (without acceptance) that he was paying for the most sudden and complete shock one could administer to a body of workers. Imagine miners and their forefathers, for hundreds of years working in the dark like moles, and then suddenly, all at once, they are working in daylight. It doesn't take much psychology, even amateur psychology, to see that that has got to be paid for; it's got to be either prepared for or paid for.

In all three cases the reaction of these hide-bound trade unionists to a new situation, to a sudden new situation, is one of demanding more money. They don't talk about pay or remuneration or wages, they talk about money—heat money, dirt money, wet money. They might have talked about shock money in the case of this pit. It *was* shock money. The colliery manager was paying for his failure, or that of his superiors, to appreciate the proper relationship between human relations and mechanical efficiency in industry.

Every employer thinks that when he transforms the conditions, and makes things much better, the men and women who work for him ought to be grateful. Well, look at the great new steel plants. They are so enormous a contrast with what went before. When the ordinary worker looks at these great, new, shining edifices and compares them with the old-fashioned steelworks, he will naturally be very suspicious of the change. The gentlemen who have built the new plants, and who go on to paint them in pastel shades, are thinking very often in terms of some eminent public figure, even a Royal figure, coming to open them. It is a recurring grievance in industry, though very seldom publicly expressed, that every time a distinguished visitor comes along, the management have the place transformed. It has been known for them to whitewash the coals. In either case, whether it is being done temporarily, for a special visit, or whether it is being done permanently, to gratify the aesthetic taste of the Public Relations Organiser, the men know that it is not they who are being consulted, and that the marvellous new conditions are not really being carried out with a view to making industry a more human place. They knew that the machine still comes first and that they still come second.

Now this may be part of our civilization. It might be the only way of running it. It was said of the early Industrial Revolution that 'things are in the saddle and ride mankind'. This may still be true. All I am suggesting is that we should look with a new eye on the reactions of trade unionists. By trade unionists I mean those stupid rank and file characters who, with all their stupidity, still control their own leaders and still dictate how the union should react to a new situation. I could have a new sub-title here, 'Digression on the Trade Union Movement's admirable refusal to conform to the Machine', but I will leave it at that just now. Let me add merely that, hard as it may be for us to admit it, these trade unionists are fellow-resisters of ours against large-scale, anonymous, chromium-plated, industrial civilization.

My next topic is the anthropologist considered as a philosophical smuggler. One anthropologist, working in one of the Western Isles, is interested mainly in the impact of 'the machine', the large scale and depersonalized mechanism of modern society, on the small 'Gemeinschaft' communities, the neighbourly communities of the Western Isles. This particular island is being invaded in all manner of ways by the economic practices of the mainland. And what I was interested to find was that not only did he assume that the final conquest of the 'Gemeinschaft' community, the old community, by the new was inevitable, but also that it was right, it was justified. This seemed to me to show the anthropologist importing into his 'objective' approach, his 'non-evaluative' approach, the belief that the kind of man who succeeds in our society is the kind of man who ought to succeed in any society.

Sooner or later the old life must go, the island ways must be submerged and the people must change their ways completely, and on the whole he thinks it is a good thing; not only because he thinks it is inevitable but because it is civilization on the march. 'Gesellschaft' is civilization. Now this is a reasonable point of view. But it is important to be clear that it conveys a value judgement. Professor Polanyi has already shown that the failure to admit this kind of transition is an occupational disease of anthropologists.

A second recent and valuable study (also unpublished) makes no such illicit transition. It is a straightforward account of people living in two kinds of district—a new housing estate, and an older district, in a smallish English city. It is important for our theme because the observer detects in both settings an apparent emotional frustration and conflict in the women in the house. He ascribed it in the first case to the special conditions of the new housing estate, tracing it to a fear that the family would be put out of the house if they didn't behave themselves and keep quiet; a fear of the mysterious powers in the Town Hall who had found them the house. Another source, he suggested, might be the absence of a varied and close associational life such as is experienced in old-established communities.

But he found the same kind of frustration and discontent in the older part of the city. There the wife's mother is just round the corner. The family has social supports of a kind which don't exist in the new housing estate. There is no fear of the landlord. But the woman of the house showed much the same kind of frustration and discontent. No conclusions are offered in the study about this, and I have no conclusions to offer. But it can be suggested that women, who as a class have benefited greatly by the liberating influences of industrial society, still don't like the disruptive effects of the greater freedom they have. This double attitude of welcome towards some of the effects of the machine, and rejection of others, is damaging to their personal stability and happiness.

The woman in the house, or the woman torn between house and outside work, is the chief contemporary victim of the tension engendered by the free mechanized society. It is a problem which affects all of us but which is particularly pressing in her case. And this suggests the point on which we should concentrate our study of 'man and the machine'.

Reflections

M. B. FOSTER

Student of Christ Church, Oxford

IN ORDER TO relate some of the topics discussed in this book,
we need a connecting thread. The thread I have chosen is this:
I am going to suggest that the things we want are of two kinds.
There are things we can get by aiming at them, and there are
things we cannot get by aiming at them. Or to put it in another way: some of the things we want are things we know
how to get, and some are things which, in that sense at any
rate, we don't know how to get. This seems to me to be illustrated in Professor Macbeath's chapter on ritual. He says there
(page 49) that ritual has its functions, beneficial results which
it produces; for example, it produces courage and confidence,
or can, among those who use it. But, he adds, 'ritual can
produce these results only if the actors consciously and deliberately aim at or intend something else'. That is to say, if you
are a primitive man, and if you believe that this kind of ritual
will make the rain fall and the crops grow, and if this is the
thing you have in mind when you chant the ritual, then as a
by-product, you will get the courage and the confidence; but
if you say 'We have outgrown this primitive state, but we want
the courage and the confidence' and you do the ritual in order
to get this, you won't get it. This is an example, it seems to me,
of the case where you cannot get the thing that you want by
aiming at it. And therefore, one is in an obvious dilemma. You
are in the position of wanting something, and yet knowing

that the attempt to get it will defeat your own end; and it seems to me that this same dilemma runs through much of Mr. Adler's chapter and Mr. John Mack's discussion of human relations in an industrial society.

Mr. Adler is concerned with the depersonalization which follows upon a market economy, and he illustrates it by the obvious example of the depersonalization of human relations in an industrial society. Now, one of the things he says is that this depersonalization can be, and is counteracted, and the relations humanized again, by the pressure of a common purpose, such as one has in war, because then exactly the same thing happens as happens with the people who believe in the ritual. If the intention of the workers and, of course, of the managers, is directed upon the common purpose of winning the war, then as a result of this, as a by-product of this, the improvement or the humanization of the workers takes place.

But supposing you say, 'Well, we don't want a war but we do want the by-product', and you then direct your attention upon producing these improved human relations, you are in the same dilemma as in the previous case. You cannot get it by trying to get it; it seems you can get it only by trying to get something else. The same deliemma is brought out in John Mack's chapter. He says, and I don't doubt it, that the mistake is that managers place increased productivity before human relations. They ought to put it the other way round; they ought to pursue the human relations and then let the increased productivity be the by-product. But that doesn't solve my dilemma, which still remains. Supposing you take the attitude which Mr. Mack recommends, supposing you say that better human relations is the thing we want, you are still in the dilemma that this doesn't seem to be a thing you can get by aiming at it. As to the way in which this thing is to be got, I don't think the dilemma is solved; but I think some light is thrown upon it by something else in Mr. Mack's remarks.

Human relations, he says, are improved only if there is on the part of the directors or the management *a genuine concern* for their improvement. This fact seems to me significant. It seems to imply that the improvement of human relations is a peculiar thing. It doesn't depend upon what is done. I don't mean that what is done is unimportant, but the essential thing, I gather, is not *what* is done but that what is done should witness to a genuine concern. The vital thing, in other words, is not the thing you can do on purpose; it is not something resulting from the action taken; it seems to follow from the genuine concern, the disinterested goodwill, to which the action taken bears witness.

But if one thinks that is true, one is left with a problem. Supposing the genuine concern is lacking; how are you to get it? How are we to get it in ourselves? It is not a question I can really start asking, because if I had not any genuine concern, I would not want it, and would not even begin to try to get it. Or, again, suppose it is lacking in some managements, in those managements which introduce the system and it fails. This is not as if some technical defect is being diagnosed. We can set about the supply of that. But supposing the thing which we diagnose to be lacking is 'genuine concern', how do you set about putting genuine concern into managements? That is the dilemma as it appears in the social sphere, but it seems to me you can see the same thing on the individual level. If one thinks of the choices and the sort of policy one adopts in the conduct of personal life, one can see the same distinction between the things one can get by trying to get them, (and then, if one fails, the thing is to try harder), and the things which cannot be got in that way at all.

As an example of the second things, the things you cannot get by trying to get them directly, let us take successful personal relations with the people we are closely connected with, the people we meet, with everybody we come across. It seems to me that this is certainly a thing we want, more than almost anything else; and yet it is one of those peculiar things which we cannot set about trying to get in the way we can set about trying to get other things. To illustrate the difference, think of the different problem which is involved in building a model house (an ideal house, or 'ideal home', as it were), and making a happy household. The first is a technical problem, the second is a problem of personal relations. What I am suggesting is that there is a difference between these two kinds of things, a difference not only of practice, in that the one is more difficult than the other, but a difference of principle. If you lack one of the things which go to the equipment of the ideal house, the remedy is to try harder and to learn more; but if the other things are lacking, those which concern the personal relations of the family in the house, it may be that these are not merely more difficult things of the same kind, but a different kind of thing. It may be that these are things which are in principle unobtainable by trying, and hence that it is no good trying to obtain them.

That is the distinction which I am suggesting as the thread, the distinction between these two kinds of things. If we are to get things of these two kinds, we have to go about getting them, it seems, in different ways. I would like to add, as a sort of appendix, something about the relation of this to science. I am going to suggest that this distinction between the things you aim at directly, and the things you cannot get by aiming at them directly, coincides with the distinction between the things which can be obtained by science and those which cannot. I am not now thinking about the nature of science as knowledge, and its relation to other kinds of knowledge.[1] I am thinking of science solely in relation to the kind of things which science is capable of *doing*. I am suggesting that things of the kind which we can get by aiming at them are the things to which we can apply science. If there are the other kind of things, these are the things to the obtaining of which science cannot be applied. I mean, to take my simple example, you can employ science to improve the house, but you cannot directly employ science to improve the human relations inside it.

This, I think—I hope I am right—would be accepted by all the contributors to this volume who have discussed this subject. It seems to me to be a point which many of them have made. But it is not a distinction which always has been made. People have thought that deficiencies in human relations can be removed by more science. That position is strikingly maintained in Dr. Barbara Wootton's book *Testament of Social Science*. She contends that what is needed is the application of social science to human problems, and that this will solve—or at least that this is the only hope of solving—the

[1] In the way in which Dr. Martin Johnson treated it.

frustrations and the difficulties an the deficiencies from which we suffer. I do not know whether she would still say that, (her book was written some years ago), but other people before her have said that the troubles of the world at the present time are due to the fact that our progress in the natural sciences has outrun our progress in the social sciences; and I have even seen it suggested that what we must do is to call a halt in the one and develop the other more vigorously, until we have redressed the balance.

Now, if the development of the social sciences means the application of scientific techniques to the social sphere, I must say this seems to me wholly mistaken. The development of the social sciences could, it seems to me, do nothing except give us another and still greater instrument of power, without giving us help in the direction of its use.

So far I have not said anything about ways to attain the kinds of things which are unattainable by direct assault, or by science, but other contributors have dealt with them. Mr. Westmann says that the whole ground and aim of human existence is to achieve a relationship of awareness to personality. And in the chapters on the religions there is mention of these kinds of ends which are not scientifically attainable, e.g., in what Professor Quispel says about Gnosis. According to the *non*-Christian form of Gnosis, he tells us, there are three classes of men—the mob of men who pursue material ends; the pious, the churchgoers; and finally the 'Gnostics', those who achieve self-knowledge and self-realization, and this is the thing supremely worth having. Now, this end which the Gnostics put before themselves, is, I think, something which rings a bell with quite a number of people. It seems to promise something which the pursuit of material ends and churchgoing do not offer. This self-knowledge and self-realization are not among the things we can get by trying. The Ancient Gnostics did not think it was. They believed that it was purely a matter of destiny. Those who have not got the divine spark cannot get it, and those who have got it cannot avoid realizing it. This self-realization which formed the central point of their beliefs, was one of the things belonging to my second class.

In Buddhism one thing is supremely important; knowledge of sorrow and the cessation of sorrow, and the Buddhist believes not only that this thing is supremely important but that we can learn how to get it. He believes that we can learn how to get it, not by science, at least not by science in the sense in which we use the word, but by a method which is non-scientific (in the modern sense). Now, certainly, the fact that the Buddhist method is not scientific *might* not in itself mean very much, because of course, Buddhism is very old and there are a great many things which previously were pursued by unscientific methods but are now obtainable by scientific ones. In fact, this is true of almost everything which is capable of technical production. Pottery, for example, used to be produced by an unscientific method, with, I do not doubt, a lot of religious elements mixed up in it; ironwork too, and almost every technical process you can think of. There was in primitive times an unscientific and probably religious way of getting the products, but this has now been replaced by a scientific way and of course the old way is discarded; it has had its day and no one can now go back to it.

Is this the case with Buddhism? Certainly Buddhism is a non-scientific method—is it a pre-scientific pursuit of something *which is in principle scientifically attainable*? I raise this question because I think it will elucidate the distinction between the things attainable by science and the things which are not. What is the end of Buddhism? Dr. Basham, in his most illuminating paper, tells us that the end, the aim which this method pursues, is the cessation of sorrow. Now, something *like* that is certainly scientifically attainable. For example, if instead of saying 'cessation of sorrow', one says 'banishment of pain', that can be and is attained scientifically. We have only to think of the science of anaesthetics, and it may well be that the science of anaesthetics is only in its beginnings. Moreover, mental pain, mental distress, also—I think I am right in saying this—can be diminished, if not banished, by brain surgery, and this is certainly scientific. Again, we cannot say how far the science of brain surgery may not go. Could we think that if these sciences progress further, they will achieve by scientific means what the Buddhist was after in his unscientific methods?

Well, Dr. Basham, I suppose, is really the person who ought to answer this. I would say: 'No', although I suppose it may have been the case (in fact, it must have been the case), that what the Buddhist was after was not clearly distinguished from cessation of pain in this sense. Nevertheless cessation of pain in this sense, if you had said to him, 'Is this what you want?' would not have been what he wanted. So that the Buddhist aim, or some element of the Buddhist aim, is something not to be achieved by science (*in principle* not to be achieved by science) but something which the Buddhist believes can be achieved by some method other than science.

I should like now to say a few words about the relation of Christianity to this theme. Christianity, if one compares it with Gnosis and Buddhism, has its own conception of a supremely worth-while thing corresponding to the 'self-realization' of Gnosis and the 'cessation of sorrow' of Buddhism. This is called in the New Testament 'inheriting the Kingdom of God', or 'eternal life'.

According to Christianity, is there a way of getting these? I would say that in Christianity there is not a *method* of getting them in the sense in which Buddhism thinks there is. It is true, of course, there is the commandment, 'Seek ye the Kingdom of God', but for Christianity—and here I may be speaking too crudely in relation to Buddhism; I do not know enough about it to be sure—there is certainly no *technique* of securing it. This makes the difference between it and the things which are scientifically attainable. You cannot obtain it; it can be had, but (this is the crucial thing), when it comes, it is given by God. This seems to me very important, the basis of the whole Christian attitude to these things. We have a part, but man's part is not to get the Kingdom of God, but something quite different; his part is what the Bible calls 'repentance and faith'. These, of course, are words and it is easy to use words not only without conveying one's meaning, but even without putting meaning into them. I do not forget the horror which Dr. Oldham feels and often expresses at the sort of glibness which accompanies the use of Christian terms. The difficulty is to bring these terms down to brass tacks. I will try to do that in a few rather haphazardly selected ways by bringing this doctrine into relation, if I can, with some of the answers given by the other doctrines.

Christianity says you cannot obtain the Kingdom of God. In this respect it differs from Buddhism, and in this respect it is like what you might call the negative views which I started off by describing. But it does not stop there. It says you cannot obtain it, the Kingdom of God, and then it makes the significant addendum—*but* God can give it. This is, it seems to me, the important thing here, to give sense to the addendum, to see what it means when it is brought down to brass tacks. Some words by Dom John Chapman quoted by Dr. Stella Churchill are relevant here: 'Don't try to make yourself good, God will see to that'. There is an *existential* difference between the kind of attitude to life expressed in saying merely 'Don't try to make yourself good', and the attitude expressed in saying 'Don't try to make yourself good, God will see to that'. If these added words really express something existential, then I think it will be true to say that it implies what the New Testament calls 'repentance and faith'. A further difference between Christianity and Buddhism is that the Christian God is not just a God who is within the universe, but a God who created the universe and who is the controller of everything that is in it. If this is 'existentially' believed, it transforms our attitude to worry. We can't *stop* worrying by trying to stop, but it is a new attitude when we cease to worry about worrying. This is something like the attitude of Job. Job in a way was overwhelmed with worry, but the fundamental thing about Job was that he knew that all the worries came from God. Nothing can exceed the exasperation and the bitterness of Job's protest; but the basic thing was that it was God whom he had to deal with all the time.

Professor Quispel makes some very illuminating remarks about the relation of Christianity to Gnosis. If you contrast the Gnostic with the Christian doctrine, two things, he observes, are fundamentally different. According to the Gnostic doctrine, the world is devilish. The Gnostic is divine, he has the divine spark, and he has to make the passage of the divine spark through the devilish world. According to the Christian, the world is good, and God made it. And secondly, whereas

according to the Gnostic, self-realization is confined to a
certain class of people, according to the Christian, salvation is
offered to all classes of people, to the materialists and even to
the churchgoers. But now, this is the important thing; it is
not that Christianity takes the two lower classes, the materialists
and the churchgoers, and then banishes the top class; it is not
as if it resigns the thing which the Gnostic thought most
valuable. The Christians claimed that Christianity is the true
Gnosis. Professor Quispel says that this claim was made by St.
Paul, and by Clement. This seems to me most illuminating
for the understanding of what Christianity is, because it means
that this self-knowledge and self-realization which the Gnostics
are after is not resigned or treated as a bad thing, or as something unimportant, but as something which is offered to the
churchgoers and the mobs. Let us think, if we may, of what
this self-knowledge and this self-realization are in the Christian
context. What is the Christian Gnosis, if one can put it like
this? Know yourself and be yourself. Now, it makes a difference what you know yourself as, or what you realize yourself
as. What we are concerned with here, I think, is a difference of
archetypes; one can understand it partly by thinking of the
difference between the Gnostic archetype and the Christian
archetype. Archetype means literally 'master pattern'; and if
one thinks of the Gnostic archetype (the picture comprising
these three classes of people and the whole cosmic view), and
of the Christian archetype on the other side—according to
what archetype are you seeking to know yourself or to realize
yourself? According to the Gnostic, you seek to know yourself
and to realize yourself as divine. According to the Christian,
you seek to know yourself and to realize yourself as a creature
of God. Of course, both expressions are symbolic; they derive
from a mythological use of language; but it makes a great
difference which you say, providing it is not merely a matter of
saying, but is, so to speak, a matter of belief. Suppose it is a
matter of existential acceptance, then which of these is at the
basis makes the whole difference to the kind of life which is
lived. The Gnostic self-knowledge and self-realization was
to know yourself as divine. Christian self-knowledge and
self-realization is to know yourself as a man. As to what this

involves, I would like to illustrate by quoting a few lines from Dietrich Bonhoeffer, the German Protestant theologian. He says (I am translating freely, but I think I am giving the sense):

> To be united with Christ means to be an actual man. The actual man can afford to be the creature that God made him; he can afford to be the man that he actually is. This puts an end to pose, hypocrisy, tension, to the necessity of being something different, something more ideal than one is.

This, if Christianity is the true Gnosis, is the true self-knowledge, not the cultivation of the divine spark; and this puts not only self-knowledge, but personal relations on a different footing. Professor Quispel says something about this also when he refers to the ethical implications of Gnosticism. For the Gnostic there was no encounter with other people. Others were a means to his self-realization. But the Christian meets others as men, and that, on this point, is the Christian doctrine. You can only know yourself as you are, and you can only meet others as men, by supernatural grace, and 'by supernatural grace' means—or at least it involves—that you cannot get it; you cannot do it by trying; but you can be given it.

In conclusion, I would like to say a word more about 'archetypes'. This conception of an archetype does throw light for me on what having a faith means, and on difference it makes whether we have one faith or another. I found in a book by Josef Pieper, a German Catholic theologican, called *The End of Time*, a description that seemed to me to illustrate very well one aspect of what an archetype is. He writes: 'I look upon things—but this reality spread out before my eyes is illuminated by a light at which I do *not* look, which is, rather, situated behind my back, but which illuminates things for my eyes only if "I believe".' You see, the archetype is something behind your back as it were, but if it is accepted it illuminates the things which are before your eyes.

This reminds me of something which Dr. Mackay says about different levels at which you can see, for example, the material word, as you can the lights of an electric advertising sign: the sign at one level is an arrangement of electric-light bulbs, but this does not prevent you from seeing it also as something else, namely, as a sentence which makes sense. But, of course, you see it as *this* only if you can read, which means that at this level you are seeing something which is really in it, but which you will see only if you have got something like the illumination which Pieper mentions. But one must not be misled by such an image into thinking it is *simply* a matter of the way in which you look at the world. What archetype is accepted makes a difference also to attitude and conduct, and I should like to see if one can make this a bit more concrete by setting side by side the picture of Christian conduct and the picture of Buddhist conduct.

One of the most interesting and attractive things, for me, in Dr. Basham's paper is the picture he gives of the Buddhist pattern, what it looks like when it is worked out in life (the master-pattern working itself out into details). He quotes Buddha's *Sermon of the Admonition to Sigala*, explaining the ethical duties of the 'Six Sides', the north and the south, the east and the west and the top and the bottom (page 88).

I propose to set side by side with that an example of the Christian pattern, taken from Paul's Sermon of the Admonition to the Romans, which I will read in the Authorized Version. (Please bear in mind, for comparison, the Buddhist admonitions). St. Paul writes: 'Let love be without dissimulation. Abhor that which is evil; cleave to that which is good. Be kindly affectioned one to another with brotherly love; in honour preferring one another; not slothful in business; fervent in spirit; serving the Lord; rejoicing in hope; patient in tribulation; continuing instant in prayer; distributing to the necessity of saints; given to hospitality; bless them which persecute you; bless and curse not. Rejoice with them that do rejoice, and weep with them that weep. Be of the same mind one toward another. Mind not high things, but condescend to men of low estate. Be not wise in your own conceits. Recompense to no man evil for evil. Provide things honest in the sight of all men. If it be possible, as much as lieth in you, live peaceably with all men. Dearly beloved, avenge not yourselves, but rather give place unto wrath; for it is written, Vengeance is mine, I will repay, saith the Lord. Therefore, if thine enemy hunger, feed him; if he thirst, give him drink: for in so doing thou shalt heap coals of fire on his head. Be not overcome of evil, but overcome evil with good.'

And on the negative side, on the side of the things which are not enjoined but forbidden, I will quote *Galatians*, chapter V. 'The works of the flesh are manifest.' (I am afraid flesh in St. Paul is a misleading word, at least I think it is misleading to our modern ears. I think I am right in saying that what Paul means by 'flesh' is not what we normally have in mind, namely the desires of the flesh as distinct from the spirit, the body as distinct from the spirit. The works of the flesh, as you will see when you hear the list, can be quite spiritual things. The flesh in St. Paul is the *man, body and spirit*, in so far as he is not united with God.) These are the works of the flesh: 'Adultery, fornication, uncleanness, lasciviousness, idolatry, witchcraft, hatred, variance, emulations, wrath, strife, seditions, heresies, envyings, murders, drunkenness, revellings, and such like: Of the which I tell you before, as I have also told you in time past, that they which do such things shall not inherit the kingdom of God.'

To compare and contrast those two pictures is something I am not capable of, and I shall not attempt it. Obviously there are similarities, obviously there are characteristic differences; these are two different patterns of life, and I am sure one would find that one could run these differences back to the differences in the archetypal beliefs. But I would like to say a word on the difference in the *status* of the ethical code in Christianity and in Buddhism. For the Buddhist, if I have understood rightly, these things are recommendations from someone who has tried them. They are like the recommendations from someone who has tried a cure, let us say, a medical cure; he has found it works, and so, if you like, he shows you what it is. It is for you to take it or leave it. I hope this is not putting it too crudely. For the Christian, also, in a sense it is, 'Take it or leave it' ('Therefore choose' says the Bible), but it is not 'Take it or leave it' quite in the same way, because the Christian way is not something which has been discovered by a man and found to work. It is a way of life laid down by God. That makes an important difference.

It is assumed, of course, by St. Paul, first, that those whom he addresses want more than anything else to inherit the Kingdom, and secondly that they do not know how to do this. This is not a thing which anybody could know but God; this is the grace, the free gift of God, God has revealed the way. Now, if it is looked upon like this, it seems to me to make irrelevant some rational criticism which is sometimes exercised on Christian morals (especially on Christian morals about sex, but it could apply equally to other things), and also, perhaps, to make irrelevant some Christian attitudes towards those who reject Christian morals. If a person say these rules are irrational, the answer surely is, 'Do you know a better way to the kingdom of God?' If he then says 'I don't want the kingdom of God', that alters the situation, and the Christian cannot quite go on talking to him as though he did want the kingdom of God. There is another thing to be done first, to make him want the kingdom of God—though this, again, is misleading, because I have been talking as though the kingdom of God is something which you can choose either to have or not to have. This leaves out something which is too big to embark upon. The other point, and the other difference in Christian belief, is that the kingdom of God is coming anyway, though it makes a great difference whether it is accepted and welcomed or whether it is rejected.